Problem-Solving in Nursing Practice

FOUNDATIONS OF NURSING SERIES

WM. C. BROWN COMPANY PUBLISHERS

ANNA KUBA
Consulting Editor

Nursing Observation
Virginia B. Byers
Monroeville, Pennsylvania

Nursing Observations of the Young Patient
Margaret A. Coffin
Boston University School of Nursing

Promotion of Physical Comfort and Safety
Valentina G. Fischer and Arlene F. Connolly
Boston University School of Nursing

Promoting Psychological Comfort
Gloria M. Francis and Barbara Munjas
Medical College of Virginia

Problem-Solving in Nursing Practice
Mae M. Johnson, Mary Lou C. Davis, and Mary Jo Bilitch

Nurse-Patient Communication
Garland K. Lewis
Catholic University of America

Working with Others for Patient Care
Grace G. Peterson
DePaul University

Teaching Function of the Nursing Practitioner
Margaret L. Pohl
Hunter College

Planning Patient Care
Lucile Lewis
Loma Linda University

Problem-Solving in Nursing Practice

Mae M. Johnson
Mary Lou C. Davis
Mary Jo Bilitch

Los Angeles Valley College

5568

WM. C. BROWN COMPANY PUBLISHERS
Dubuque, Iowa

Library of Congress Catalog Card Number: 77—106947

ISBN 0—697—05531—0

Third Printing, 1971

Printed in the United States of America

Nursing today is experiencing new developments in basic knowledge and practices. The appearance of new concepts, along with greater diversification in health care facilities, has created a demand for nurses equipped with the knowledge and abilities to promote health, prevent disease and injury, and care and comfort the helpless and sick.

The **Foundations of Nursing Series** is in response to the need for new educational material in the field. The individual volumes in this Series include the knowledge and skills now being incorporated into modern nursing practices. This Series offers both the student and teacher flexibility of subject matter, as well as authoritative writing in each text area. Although the individual titles are self-contained, collectively they cover the major subjects, as discussed in introductory courses.

Dedicated to the memory of

Mary Jo Bilitch

PREFACE

This book presents an introduction to the process of problem-solving as it is used in the practice of nursing. It offers a discussion of each step in the process: assessment, problem identification, problem statement, decision, action, and evaluation. It is intended for use in vocational, diploma, associate, and baccalaureate degree programs, in-service programs, and for individual practitioners who wish to review the subject and improve their understanding and use of the problem-solving process.

The need for a more complete presentation of this subject than is ordinarily included in textbooks on nursing has been voiced by students, practitioners, and instructors. In recent years the nursing profession has given emphasis to the need for a more scientific approach to patient care by nurse practitioners. The achievement of continuity of nursing care is a goal that has been given high priority. Much time and effort has been expended to develop the written nursing care plan as one means by which continuity can be attained. Ability to use the problem-solving process is essential to the development of the plan for nursing care. When the nurse has learned to use this method of thinking in the practice of nursing, there is increased awareness of the nature of the plan and its rationale. This facilitates its translation into verbal form for communication between all nursing personnel caring for a given patient.

Although the book offers an examination of each step, greater emphasis is given to assessment and problem identification. In fact, it might well be considered a book on problem-finding. The authors believe these to be the areas of greatest need. Experience reveals that failure to meet patient needs occurs most frequently because of failure to correctly identify the problem. If the patient problem can be recognized, then the nurse's problem or problems can be better identified. This book makes a sincere effort to differentiate between the patient problem and the nursing problem, an area which is not clear in many publications.

Improvement in nursing care can be attained by assisting nurses to develop the mental process by which they collect and analyze patient information and identify patient problems. This process is for the most part invisible. One cannot look into the minds of those experienced in this type of thinking and observe how facts are accumulated and sorted and how conclusions are drawn. This book endeavors to provide students and nurses with a look at the workings of the mind in the practice of nursing.

An attempt has been made to offer an easy-to-understand approach. Scientific terminology has been kept to a minimum. When contemporary terms have been used, they are defined or explained. Every effort has been made to carry the reader in logical steps to a conclusion, and it is highly recommended that it be used in its chronological sequence for best results. By use of examples, exercises, suggested readings, and line drawings, the book is also meant to be enjoyed.

ACKNOWLEDGMENTS

Acknowledgments are difficult at best, and someone who should receive our gratitude is bound to be inadvertently missed. Several members of the nursing faculty at Los Angeles Valley College have been most helpful, and an especially warm "thank you" goes to Mrs. Patsy Sapra for her comments and constructive criticism. Since problem-solving in nursing practice has been in use by the nursing students in our program, they, too, deserve credit for their candid reactions and contributions. Certainly family members are always due a word of appreciation for their moral support. A sincere "thank you" goes to Miss Virginia Carew for her helpful review, to Joyce Watson, our typist, and, of course, to Chris Kinsch, who contributed our line drawings.

MAE M. JOHNSON
MARY LOU C. DAVIS

CONTENTS

Chapter 1

Problem-Solving—An Overview

Man has always recognized and solved problems. It is his capacity for mentally perceiving and storing information about himself and his environment and his ability in reflective thinking that enables him to do this. When he uses these abilities in a conscious, organized manner, we say he is using "the process of problem-solving" or "the problem-solving approach." Matheny, et al, states:

> "If we take this ordinary reflective thought process as a base, we can proceed to sharpen and define certain aspects and easily reach what is technically called the scientific method, or the problem-solving approach. Taken by themselves, the steps of the problem-solving approach involve ordinary mental activities carried out daily by every person. Taken collectively, they amount to the most dynamic technique devised by man to know and to control our environment."[1]

You have been using this process to solve problems all of your life. As an infant you felt uncomfortable. You recognized that your need for comfort was not being met, that is, you had the problem "discomfort." You cried (you took action) and someone relieved your discomfort (solution was achieved). At home or in social situations, as a student or as an employee, you have used this process to recognize and solve problems. Therefore, what follows will not be entirely new to you. The objective here is to examine this process and to clarify its components so that you can increase your skill and, as a nurse, use it to help patients solve their physical and mental health problems.

---

[1]Ruth Matheny, et al., *Fundamentals of Patient Centered Nursing* (St. Louis: The C. V. Mosby Co., 1964), p. 26,

PROBLEMS AND PROBLEM-SOLVERS

Man is a creature with many needs which require fulfillment if he is to attain and maintain his physical and psychological equilibrium. Frequently factors develop in his internal and external environment which interfere with the attainment and maintenance of this fulfillment. When needs are not met, there are problems. Man must do something to solve these problems or he will ultimately perish. Man's world demands "that he adapt to it, manipulate it, change it, and create in it."[2] In so doing he prevents or eliminates those factors which threaten his physical and mental health. To do this, he must learn what his essential needs are, what kinds of problems can develop in various circumstances, and what means are available for avoiding or solving the problem.

Most of the time people want to and are able to control their own lives. They keep alert to dangers and attempt to avoid them. They come to recognize unfulfilled needs. They take action to meet such needs and in the process are solving problems.

There are times, however, when people are unable to identify their problems or solve those which they do recognize. They may lack the physical, emotional, spiritual, social, or economic capability. They may lack the expert skills which are necessary to carry out the components of the solution. In these situations, man turns to his fellowman for assistance. He seeks a problem-solver.

Society, through education, prepares people with the various skills needed. We find, therefore, in our complex modern society people who are skilled in such diverse pursuits as that of the businessman, the lawyer, the physician, the psychologist, and so on. Each person offers the skills he has to the other members of society who need them.

Within most occupational groups there are those who are skilled at identifying the problem and developing a plan for solving it, and those who are skilled at performing the tasks or actions which solve the problem. The civil engineer, for example, may observe a freeway problem that is snarling traffic and devise a plan for solving it. The pile driver, the road grader, the cement mixer, and other such workers will then be brought to coordinate their efforts toward the objective. These people will, of course, encounter and solve many problems in the course of each day's work. They will be the solvers of *their own* problems and ultimately they will share in having solved the full problem. They were not, however, charged with the responsibility of identifying the problem and devising the plan. They were not hired as solver of the whole problem.

---

[2]Ruth Matheny, et al., *op. cit.*

In some occupational situations the same person may identify the problem, formulate and carry out a plan of action. A mechanic hired to repair your car is an example. He looks for and identifies problems, then resolves the situation with skill and experience.

THE PROBLEM-SOLVING PROCESS

Very briefly the process may be outlined as follows:

1. Encountering a problem or situation in which you discover a problem.
2. Assessing the problem or situation, that is, collecting and analyzing the data in connection with it.
3. Identifying the exact nature of the problem.
4. Deciding a plan of action.
5. Carrying out the plan.
6. Evaluating the plan and the new situation.

Each of these steps will be discussed more fully.

If you have not as yet had an opportunity to study how man perceives himself and his world, and how he thinks and reasons, you should do so now. At least a rudimentary background is necessary before you can truly understand how this process is adapted for use by nursing, or by any other occupation. Psychology, logic, and research texts are replete with information on this subject. (See bibliography for suggestions.)

THE NURSE AND PROBLEM-SOLVING

Nursing is one of the occupations that members of our society turn to for assistance in recognizing and solving their mental and physical health problems. Within the nursing world there are those who identify and formulate plans for patient care and those who perform the tasks involved. The registered nurse does the former and as one of her most important roles she may then carry out the total plan or only those parts which require the actions she alone has the skill to perform. She may delegate various phases of the plan to other members of the nursing team—the licensed vocational nurse, nursing student, aide, orderly, surgical technician, and/or the psychiatric technician. These people, like the workers on a highway plan, will solve many of their own problems and will ultimately share in the solution of the patient's problem. This is not to say that some other member of the team *never* identifies or solves a patient problem. Experienced team members, who have also developed keen powers of observation, quite often detect a problem and, in addition, are able to make suggestions for its correction. In the last analysis, however, it is the registered nurse who is held accountable for the patient's welfare and who usually identifies the problem, formulates a plan of care, and evaluates the results.

THE COMPONENTS OF NURSING PRACTICE

It is generally accepted that there are a number of component attitudes, skills, and abilities which make up nursing practice. The following are representative.

In order to practice nursing safely the nurse must be able to

1. Apply knowledge from the various sciences.
2. Perform "Procedures" (those acts approved for use by nurses, for the solution of patients' physical problems).
3. Observe.
4. Communicate.
5. Work with others.
6. Teach.
7. Manage (plan, direct, evaluate).

Recently, the ability to identify and solve problems has been added.

It seems to us, however, that the seven activities listed above are the very components of this process called "Problem-Solving." The postulate is, therefore, that the practice of nursing is essentially the practice of problem-solving. It differs from other problem-solving occupations only in the type of problems met, the acts which are its province to perform and the ways in which it utilizes the skills it shares with other occupations.

A COMPARISON

Look at the phases of the problem-solving process and the skills required to accomplish each phase.

Phases of the Problem-Solving Process	*Skills Necessary*
Assessment—collecting and Analyzing data	Application of knowledge Observation Communication Working with others
Statement of problem	Communication Working with others
Deciding a Plan	Application of knowledge Planning Working with others

Carrying out (testing) the plan	Performance of procedures Knowledge of communication techniques Observation Directing Teaching Working with others
Evaluation of plan and its results	Evaluation Observation Communication Working with others

It appears that the very skills which are used in the problem-solving process are the same as those stated above as skills of nursing practice.

WHY ALL THE EMPHASIS ON PROBLEM-SOLVING?

Why then, you may ask, is the field of nursing making all this "fuss" about problem-solving? Why are nurse educators building whole curriculums around this concept? Why are nursing service administrators revising job classifications and making employee assignments, promotions, and salary scales commensurate with ability in problem-solving? Why are nursing texts devoting space to the discussion of this subject? Why are nursing publications doing likewise?

We think the answer to these questions is that it is now being more fully recognized that the process known as problem-solving gives organization and direction to the various and distinct elements of nursing practice. It is the sum of its parts and, as such, constitutes a technique in itself. As Matheny says, "a dynamic technique." Furthermore, the authors believe:

1. That with this approach patient needs can be more thoroughly assessed and plans more effectively made to meet them;
2. That this approach focuses the nurse's thinking on the *individual* rather than the *tasks* involved in his care; and
3. That it facilitates the preparation and use of the written nursing care plan.

CAN PROBLEM-SOLVING BE TAUGHT? CAN IT BE LEARNED? ARE THERE DEGREES OF COMPETENCY?

It is known that skills necessary for problem-solving can be taught. There should, therefore, be little doubt that one can be led to the study and exploration of the various phases of the problem-solving process.

This, in turn, should enable one to arrive at a better understanding of the mental activities involved and how the process can serve as a vehicle for the application of the skills of one's practice.

We have postulated that increasing the nurse's understanding of the problem-solving process enhances the competency with which she uses inherent skills. Competency with which the nurse performs the skills of her practice will influence her ability to identify and solve problems. The two are inseparable and completely dependent on one another.

The process used to recognize and solve patient problems is the same, regardless of the talents of the persons using it or the situation in which it is utilized, but the competency with which the process is used is definitely dependent on these two factors. The nurse with the largest amount of knowledge and the greatest ability to apply it will do the best job of providing nursing service when she (1) observes, (2) communicates, (3) works with others, (4) teaches and manages. She will be the nurse who will best use the process of problem-solving. The quantity and quality of the individual nurse's education and experience and her innate capacity to profit from both will determine both her ability to study and to learn the process of problem-solving and the requisite skills.

Nurse administrators and educators must analyze the nursing situations in their communities, decide what degree of competency is required to meet them, prepare the necessary personnel, and employ them according to their abilities. Perhaps the most critical need is to devise valid and reliable methods for measuring competency in nursing skills.

NURSE: ONE IMAGE OR MANY

Until recent years, let us say until about twenty years ago, there was basically one kind of nurse practitioner. There was, likewise, in the not too distant past, one kind of medical practitioner. Even when the practitioner devoted his or her hours of work to one specific type of patient, the skills with which he practiced were fundamentally the same. If his degree of competency exceeded that of another practitioner, it was usually due to his individual capacities and aptitudes and his motivation to study and perfect his skills.

World War II spawned many technological advances and the ensuing years have seen spectacular changes in health care. Knowledge of physical and mental illness, their causes and the therapeutic treatment have expanded. The field of health occupations has likewise expanded. Medical practitioners realized that it was impossible to be expert in all phases of modern knowledge and technique. The medical profession found it necessary to develop different levels of practitioners. Some remained general practitioners. Others prepared themselves by education and practice to become experts in certain types of clinical practice. This same phenomenon has taken place in such occupations as engineering, teaching, and law.

Nursing too has been affected by the scientific and technical advances of the past half century. Medical practice in the agencies which employ the nurse creates a myriad of patient care situations. Nursing finds that it too must have a general practitioner and a specialist. This concept and these categories are not as yet clearly defined, but they have been introduced and they are going through research and experimentation. They will be a part of your future. We think we can also safely predict that among the significant differences between the two levels, (in addition to education), will be the *ability* of the practitioner to use the problem-solving process and the *complexity* of the patient situations and patient problems to which she will be assigned.

NURSING TERMINOLOGY

Language is the method by which people communicate. Many occupational groups have sort of a language or "jargon" by which they are identified in much the same way as teenagers, and certain social groups have a language of their own. Some of the words become definite, scientific terminology and become a part of the language as a whole. Other words or groups of words serve for a period of time to describe prevalent and useful concepts. They may remain if the concept remains or fade out as the concept changes or disappears. They are often difficult to define because the concept which they represent is difficult to define. There are many such terms abroad in nursing today. In the hope of facilitating communication with the reader, an attempt has been made to define a few terms which are related to the subject of the book.

Nurse: Unless otherwise qualified the term refers to a registered nurse without distinguishing between technical and professional. (The text is addressed to both the practicing nurse and the nursing student. Since the student is learning to think and act as a nurse, it was decided to speak of her as a nurse rather than nursing student in most cases. The definition in no way intends to exclude the Licensed Practical or Vocational Nurse or student since problem-solving is also included in their care of patients.)

Health Team: A group of workers in the health occupations who are working together under the leadership of the physician to render health services to a patient.

Nursing Team: A group of nursing personnel who are working together under a designated leader and working toward the achievement of specified objectives for the care of a given patient. The fact that a number of people are assigned to care for a patient does not in and of itself constitute "a team" in the sense in which the word is used in this book. If the word "team" is used in relation to a hospital or an agency which renders 24 hour nursing service then the word "team" includes the nursing personnel on all three shifts.

Process of Problem-Solving: The fundamental series of steps by which a patient problem is found and alleviated or eliminated. No attempt is made to define various degrees of competency in the use of the *process*. It is believed that the process is the same regardless of the competencies of the person using it.

Need: Those tangible and intangible items (requirements, essentials, necessities) which the human being must have in satisfactory amounts in order to attain and maintain physical and psychological homeostasis.

Patient Behavior: Any sign, symptom, act, or response made by the body as a whole or by a part of the body or the actions and responses made by the total person.

Patient Problem: A disturbance or a danger of a disturbance in physical or psychological need balance.

Nursing Assessment: The gathering of information by the nurse or nursing team about the patient's physical and psychological needs in order to determine the patient's problems.

Nursing History: A written record of the information gathered by the nurse or nursing team.

Nursing Diagnosis: A statement of the patient problem which has been identified by the nurse from the information gathered; the conclusion drawn from the information.

Nursing Problem: The question which must be answered by the nurse or nursing team in order to solve the patient problem; the goals, aims, or objectives which the nurse or nursing team must attain in order to prevent, alleviate, or eliminate the patient problem.

Problem Solution: A means which effectively prevents, alleviates, or eliminates the patient problem. The means may be dependent on a physician's written order or may be initiated independently by a nursing order.

Nursing Order: The instructions regarding patient care given to nursing personnel by the nurse delegated to plan and direct the patient's nursing care. These instructions may be written or verbal.

Nursing Care Plan: A statement or outline of the nursing problems and the nursing measures which will be used to effect a solution to the patient's problems. It may be made known to those involved in written form or by discussion. It may deal with one or many problems.

ENCOUNTERING THE PATIENT SITUATION

The nurse encounters the patient and his situation in an infinite variety of ways. Obviously it would be impossible to describe them all. For the benefit of the reader who has had little or no patient contact, let us cite a few examples. The nurse may be assigned to the care of a certain person, may receive an extensive report on his illness, and be given a complete description of his situation. She may then elect a specific time and place to meet with the patient and do so. She encountered the patient as soon as the discussion began. On the other hand, the nurse may simply "run into" the patient. She is going down the corridor and as she passes his room he calls, "Nurse, can you come here for a minute and help me?" In this case, she may know nothing whatsoever about the patient when she meets him. Most of the time, however, the circumstances of the encounter fall somewhere between these two extremes.

Who and Where Is the Patient?

For the beginning student and also for the practitioner who has worked in only one kind of health agency, it is necessary to point out that patients are found in a wide variety of health care agencies and frequently in their own homes. It is especially important to realize that a large number of patients are not in general hospitals and are not in a bed. In fact, an increasingly large number of those patients who are in general hospitals are not confined to bed much of the time. Hence, we hear the term "patient-side nursing" rather than "bedside nursing."

The patient may be found in a hospital or at home, in a doctor's office or clinic, in a school, industrial or business plant, on the battlefield or on a troop ship; in the United States, or France, or Africa, or India. He is anyone who has a physical or mental health problem and who seeks the services of a doctor and other workers in the paramedical occupations.

Regardless of where the patient is located, as soon as the nurse encounters the patient situation, she focuses on the patient and his needs. "Are his needs being met?" she asks herself. "Is there a problem?" or "Is there a reasonable chance of a problem developing?"

Finding the Problem

There are different ways of encountering problems. You may "happen" upon the problem, the problem may be brought to your attention by someone else, or you may consciously set out to discover the problem. In other words, the problem may come to you or you may go to the problem. If the bank calls you and says you are overdrawn, you know what the problem is. On the other hand, you may review your account and discover that you have made an error in calculation and are overdrawn.

The same sort of thing occurs in nursing. The patient may call you and tell you that he cannot void, that his bladder feels full and he is uncomfortable. Or, you may be making "rounds" and while at his bedside examine his abdomen, note slight distention of the bladder plus signs of discomfort and *discover* that he cannot void.

Preventing Problems

In addition to discovering problems, the nurse has a serious responsibility to prevent problems. Prevention can be a goal of the problem-solving method just as is alleviation and solution.

Unless the problem has been brought to your attention, you are on the look out for a problem or the possibility of a problem as soon as you encounter a patient. You are aware that you have a situation in which there is the likelihood of an obscure, or, at least, a not-too-obvious problem or a situation in which a problem could develop if action is not taken to prevent it.

You do this often in your own lives. You visit the doctor and dentist at regular intervals to find out if you have a health problem or to detect one early if one is developing. You take your car to the service station periodically to have it checked. When you visit Johnny's teacher to discuss his progress, review an employee's work, or talk with the college counselor about your program, you are assessing a situation, that is, you are looking for a problem or the possibility of one which in itself may be regarded as a problem.

You may or may not encounter a problem, nevertheless this is a normal activity of life. We *do* look for problems. *It is certainly better to anticipate and prevent a problem than to try to eliminate one.*

Assessment

Whether the problem comes to you or you to the problem, it is necessary to gather information. This is the first step in the diagnostic phase. *Assessment is defined as the purposeful gathering of pertinent information and the analysis of the data gathered.*

If the problem comes to you, you have a fairly specific idea of what the problem is and the assessment will probably be brief. Even if you have only a general idea of the problem, you have a head start. Most likely you will quickly be able to add the facts you need. If you have had prior experiences with the same type of problem in the same type of situation, it may require only a moment or two of reflection and analysis to be reasonably sure you have correctly identified the specific problem. If you are out looking for problems the assessment period may take a longer time—minutes or even years—depending on the complexity of the situation and the ramifications involved.

Examining the Data

The objective of your assessment has been to gather information upon which to base a conclusion. The objective of the examination is to determine if the quantity and quality of your information is satisfactory. In other words, do you have enough of the right kind of information? Have you separated fiction from fact? Have you clarified words and concepts? How reliable were the sources of your information? Have you guarded against bias and prejudice?

As the nurse becomes more skilled in data gathering, she tends to recognize information which is relevant to the problem. Actually gathering the information and examining it often takes place simultaneously: you gather a fact, examine its value, and keep or discard it accordingly.

Interpretation of Data and Drawing a Conclusion

This is probably the most crucial step in the whole process. If data are misinterpreted the consequences can be grave. Interpretation involves making relationships between the facts gathered and drawing a conclusion through the process of deduction or induction.

Both examination of the information and the interpretation are largely mental activities and as such cannot be easily observed and imitated. Therefore, they are difficult to teach and difficult to learn. Probably the best way to learn how to do this is by doing the "thinking" out loud with another more experienced person. The nurse practitioner or student frequently does this with the instructor, supervisor, or the clinical specialist, if one is available. Together they evaluate the information, keep what is useful, discard what is irrelevant, draw relationships, and arrive at a conclusion. The conclusion will be the identification of the problem. This is what is sometimes referred to as making a nursing diagnosis. The conclusion may also be that NO problem exists. In some cases you find that you do not have enough information to identify the problem, in which case you will return for further assessment.

If the problem is going to require the action of the nursing team and/or the patient then it must be put into words which express it as clearly as possible.

Deciding a Plan of Action

The more specifically the problem is defined and the clearer it is stated, the easier it will be to make plans to solve it. The plan will depend on the nature and cause of the problem, the urgency of the situation, and the resources (of supplies, equipment, and personnel) available.

Sometimes there will be several possible courses that could be taken. The value and possible results of each will have to be considered and a decision finally made.

Testing the Plan

Having made a decision you now act on it. This is the only true way to determine if your decision is correct and your plan effective. As the plan is put into motion (by the nurse, the nursing team, or the patient) the nurse notes and records the responses obtained. If the problem or the plan is complex, it may be necessary to evaluate each step of the plan and hold discussions with the people involved.

Evaluation

The authors spent much time discussing whether this phase should be called "evaluation of the plan" or "evaluation of the patient and his situation." The final decision became simply "evaluation." It is the improvement of the patient's situation that is the ultimate objective. In the process of evaluating this, the plan itself is critically examined. This is where you determine whether or not you made a wise decision. The overall effectiveness of the plan is evaluated as well as the effectiveness of the various steps within the plan. One also looks for factors that influenced the success or failure of the plan.

This phase may prove to be the most difficult and it is all too frequently neglected. Evaluating our decisions and actions is very much akin to evaluating ourselves. Self-evaluation requires a certain objectivity, a strong ego, and the ability to accept responsibility for one's own actions. This is not always easy to do. If success occurs we are sure we masterminded it. If failure occurs we are sure it was due to factors beyond our control. In both cases, it is usually a mixture of the two. The objective of the evaluation phase is to find out whether or not the goal was achieved *and why*. It is just as valuable to find out what caused success as to find out what caused failure.

"All's Well That Ends Well"

If prevention of a problem has not been possible, then we seek to alleviate or eliminate it. A solution is the desired goal of problem-solving. Semantically speaking, the word solution itself usually implies that the disturbing element has been eliminated. This, too, may not be entirely true. Alleviation to a point of lessening the severity, duration, or impact of the problem may be the only solution possible. Sometimes an answer or an explanation is offered as a possible solution but unfortunately this does not always bring complete satisfaction. For purposes of academic discussion this may be "well and good" but in reality people are concerned with results. The more concrete the results, the more satisfied they are. Therefore, when we speak of solution in the actual practice of nursing we are talking about the elimination of the problem or the alleviation of it.

AN ILLUSTRATION

Let us take an example from everyday life, view it in the various ways stated above, and examine your *modus operandi.*

The Situation

The situation consists of you and your home. One of your important needs is SAFETY. In relation to the situation you know (1) what constitutes a satisfactory standard of safety for yourself and your home; (2) what factors may endanger your safety; and (3) what factors may interfere with your ability to meet this need.

Assessment of the Situation

In the normal course of your daily activities you will be on the lookout for anything that could threaten your safety. From time to time you assess your situation to be sure there are no dangers and no hidden problems. Perhaps there comes a time when there is a long, hot, dry spell. At this time you would be more conscious of the fact that fire is a potential danger so you would specifically look for signs of fire or any factors which could increase the danger.

Discovery of a Problem

Before leaving for work one morning you make a final check of the house (assessing). Mentally, you run down a checklist: Did I turn off the stove? Did I disconnect the electric coffee pot? Did I put out that last cigarette? Did I lock the back door? You glance in the bedroom and there see a fire in the wastebasket (from that last cigarette you left on the edge of the ashtray).

Appearance of a Problem

Suppose, on the other hand, you are not even thinking about your safety. Your husband has misplaced some important papers and you are engaged in a frantic search to find them. Nevertheless, your need for safety is still there, inherent in the situation. You are simply not out looking for problems in the area at this time. The problem could appear in one of two ways: one of the children might run in shouting, "Mom, there's fire in the wastebasket," or, while searching for your husband's papers (that is, working on another problem), you could "happen upon" the fire in the bedroom.

Assessment of the Problem

Once you find the problem you may need to gather a little more information. In this particular case, probably very little. You can see at a glance that it is confined to the wastebasket, that the main fuel is paper. If the problem were more complex you might have to determine location, size, duration, cause, and ramifications. You might even have to call on someone else to help you. As information accumulates in your mind you are analyzing each fact. "Yes, that makes sense," "No, that can't be right." And so on.

Interpretation of Data and Identification of the Problem

In just a matter of seconds your mind has absorbed the fire, the facts about it, interpreted the facts, and clearly defined the problem. "Hey," you call, "there's a little fire in the wastebasket here in the bedroom." (The problem is identified and stated.)

Deciding on a Plan of Action

Immediately you select from your store of knowledge an action that you believe will solve the problem. Perhaps you have two or three possibilities in mind. You make a decision.

Testing the Plan

You dash into the bathroom, get some water, and throw it on the fire. If water were not easily accessible, you might throw on a blanket to cut off the oxygen. If you felt your efforts were inadequate, you would call the fire department.

Evaluation

Almost simultaneously with your actions and observations you begin to examine the value of your actions and the results you are obtaining. If the actions are not getting the results you wish, you can choose one of your alternate plans. In the case of the fire it would be very easy to do this. Many times in life it is not so easy to determine the value of our actions. It may mean studying human behavior or a situation slowly and painstakingly over a long period of time.

When you have had an opportunity to evaluate your actions and determine the degree to which the problem has been alleviated or eliminated, the whole process starts over. You are now ready to assess the newly-created situation.

The situation is surely so familiar to all readers that you can readily see that the whole process from the beginning to end would not take more than five minutes. True, this is an exceedingly simple problem. It was chosen precisely for that reason. There are several important concepts to be realized from this illustration.

SUMMARY

The *process* of problem-solving is not difficult. The situation and the problem may be complex, the action chosen may be difficult or complicated, the overall plan may be extensive, but the *process* is the same and can be used in any situation.

There are many nursing situations which are almost as simple and almost as quickly solved. Pain, discomfort, thirst, and hunger are often quickly recognized and eliminated.

This is largely a mental process. With experience you will do it so quickly and easily that you will not be able to say where one step ends and the next begins. Unless it is necessary to explain all or part of the situation to another, it will all be done silently.

It does lead naturally toward statement of the problem and the making of plans. It is, therefore, well suited for use in nursing where so frequently there is a team of personnel caring for a group of patients and a written Care Plan is almost a necessity if communication is to be facilitated and continuity of care is to be achieved.

If the process is studied and practiced it will create habits of thinking that will serve through a lifetime. This "good" habit, in times of stress, will safeguard against that all too frequent "bad" habit of jumping to a conclusion and hastily selecting a stereotyped answer.

One may be working on several problems at the same time. One may be working on one complex problem for one patient while working on several simple problems for another patient. The nurse may be in the solution phase of one problem and at the same time be assessing the situation of another patient. The beginning student may be expected to recognize one simple problem and select and carry out one simple solution, whereas an expert practitioner may be expected to recognize many complex problems for a number of patients and select from a myriad of possible solutions those which will best eliminate the problems.

The degree to which one can identify and solve problems is dependent on the extent of one's knowledge about patient problems and methods of solution and one's ability to carry out these actions. One cannot apply knowledge one does not have. Realization of this fact should motivate the student and practitioner to use every possible opportunity to increase their knowledge and skills.

Suggested Reading

Dewey, John. *How We Think*. Boston: D. C. Heath and Company, 1933.

Field, Minna. *Patients Are People*. Columbia University Press, 1958, 2nd ed.

Krech, David and Crutchfield, Richard S. *Elements of Psychology*. New York: Alfred A. Knopf, 1968.

Munn, Norman L. *Introduction to Psychology*. Boston: Houghton Mifflin Company, 1962.

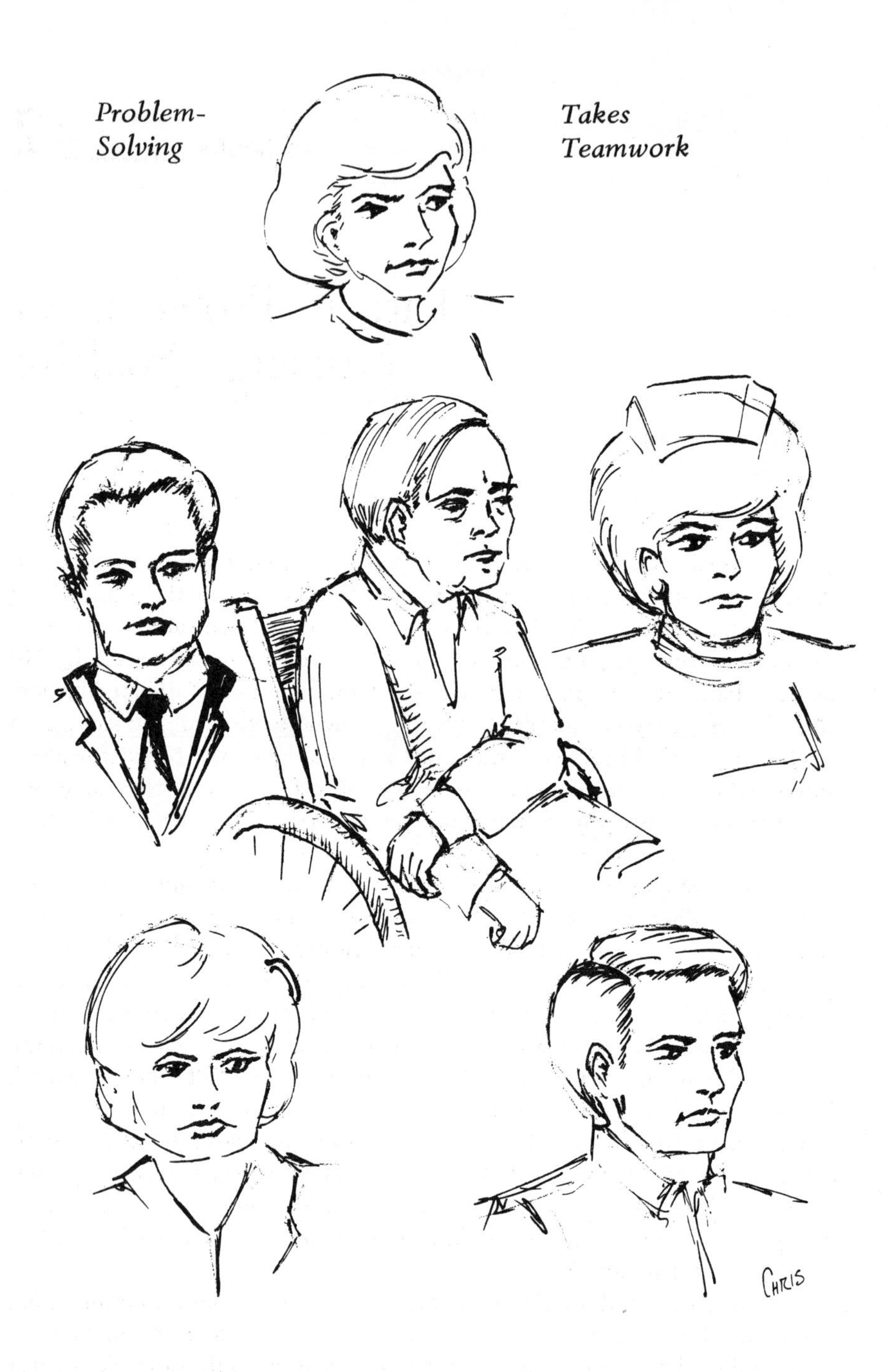
Problem-Solving
Takes Teamwork
CHRIS

SUMMARY

The *process* of problem-solving is not difficult. The situation and the problem may be complex, the action chosen may be difficult or complicated, the overall plan may be extensive, but the *process* is the same and can be used in any situation.

There are many nursing situations which are almost as simple and almost as quickly solved. Pain, discomfort, thirst, and hunger are often quickly recognized and eliminated.

This is largely a mental process. With experience you will do it so quickly and easily that you will not be able to say where one step ends and the next begins. Unless it is necessary to explain all or part of the situation to another, it will all be done silently.

It does lead naturally toward statement of the problem and the making of plans. It is, therefore, well suited for use in nursing where so frequently there is a team of personnel caring for a group of patients and a written Care Plan is almost a necessity if communication is to be facilitated and continuity of care is to be achieved.

If the process is studied and practiced it will create habits of thinking that will serve through a lifetime. This "good" habit, in times of stress, will safeguard against that all too frequent "bad" habit of jumping to a conclusion and hastily selecting a stereotyped answer.

One may be working on several problems at the same time. One may be working on one complex problem for one patient while working on several simple problems for another patient. The nurse may be in the solution phase of one problem and at the same time be assessing the situation of another patient. The beginning student may be expected to recognize one simple problem and select and carry out one simple solution, whereas an expert practitioner may be expected to recognize many complex problems for a number of patients and select from a myriad of possible solutions those which will best eliminate the problems.

The degree to which one can identify and solve problems is dependent on the extent of one's knowledge about patient problems and methods of solution and one's ability to carry out these actions. One cannot apply knowledge one does not have. Realization of this fact should motivate the student and practitioner to use every possible opportunity to increase their knowledge and skills.

Suggested Reading

Dewey, John. *How We Think*. Boston: D. C. Heath and Company, 1933.

Field, Minna. *Patients Are People*. Columbia University Press, 1958, 2nd ed.

Krech, David and Crutchfield, Richard S. *Elements of Psychology*. New York: Alfred A. Knopf, 1968.

Munn, Norman L. *Introduction to Psychology*. Boston: Houghton Mifflin Company, 1962.

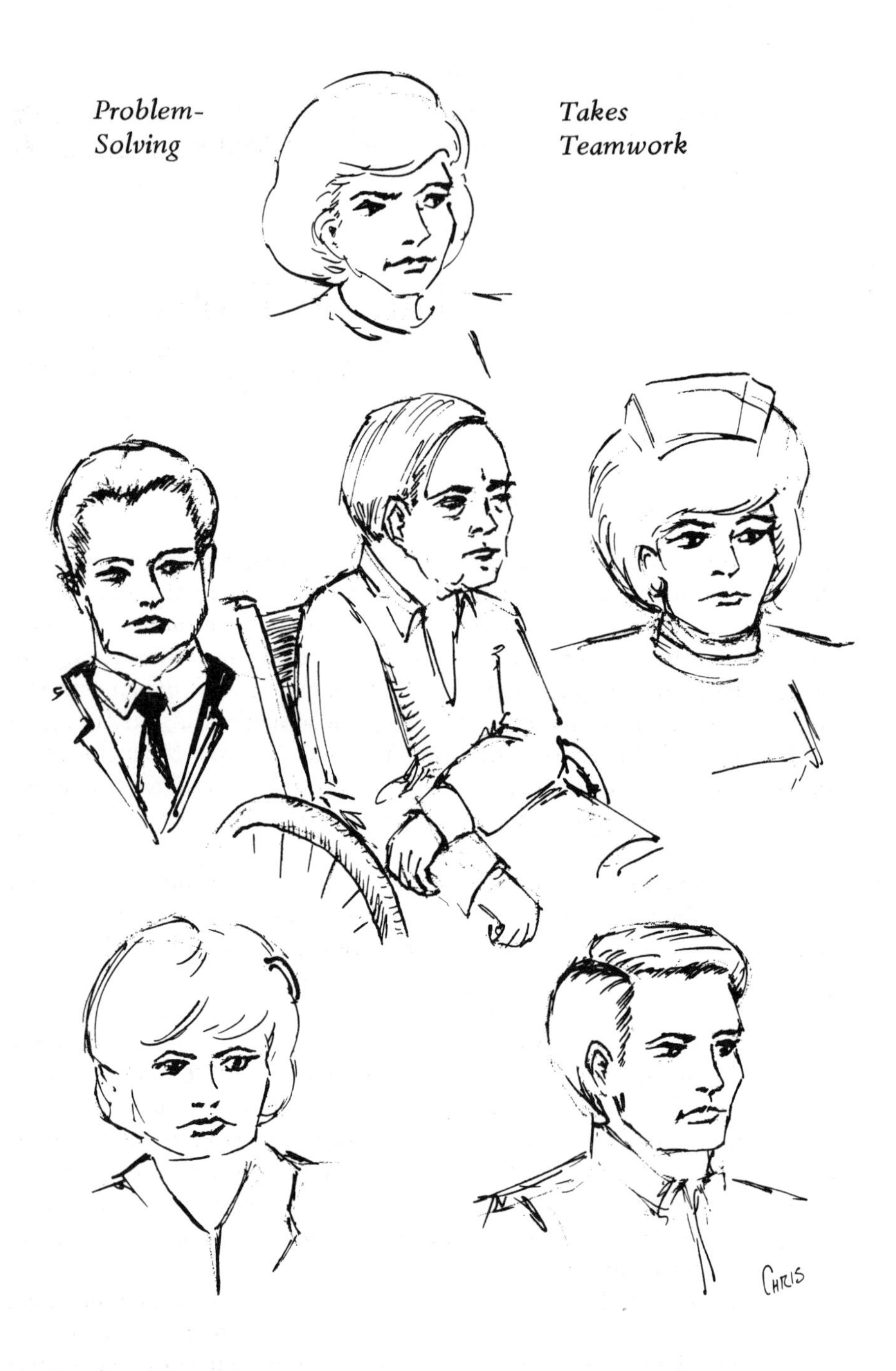

Problem-Solving Takes Teamwork

SUMMARY

The *process* of problem-solving is not difficult. The situation and the problem may be complex, the action chosen may be difficult or complicated, the overall plan may be extensive, but the *process* is the same and can be used in any situation.

There are many nursing situations which are almost as simple and almost as quickly solved. Pain, discomfort, thirst, and hunger are often quickly recognized and eliminated.

This is largely a mental process. With experience you will do it so quickly and easily that you will not be able to say where one step ends and the next begins. Unless it is necessary to explain all or part of the situation to another, it will all be done silently.

It does lead naturally toward statement of the problem and the making of plans. It is, therefore, well suited for use in nursing where so frequently there is a team of personnel caring for a group of patients and a written Care Plan is almost a necessity if communication is to be facilitated and continuity of care is to be achieved.

If the process is studied and practiced it will create habits of thinking that will serve through a lifetime. This "good" habit, in times of stress, will safeguard against that all too frequent ""bad" habit of jumping to a conclusion and hastily selecting a stereotyped answer.

One may be working on several problems at the same time. One may be working on one complex problem for one patient while working on several simple problems for another patient. The nurse may be in the solution phase of one problem and at the same time be assessing the situation of another patient. The beginning student may be expected to recognize one simple problem and select and carry out one simple solution, whereas an expert practitioner may be expected to recognize many complex problems for a number of patients and select from a myriad of possible solutions those which will best eliminate the problems.

The degree to which one can identify and solve problems is dependent on the extent of one's knowledge about patient problems and methods of solution and one's ability to carry out these actions. One cannot apply knowledge one does not have. Realization of this fact should motivate the student and practitioner to use every possible opportunity to increase their knowledge and skills.

Suggested Reading

DEWEY, JOHN. *How We Think*. Boston: D. C. Heath and Company, 1933.

FIELD, MINNA. *Patients Are People*. Columbia University Press, 1958, 2nd ed.

KRECH, DAVID and CRUTCHFIELD, RICHARD S. *Elements of Psychology*. New York: Alfred A. Knopf, 1968.

MUNN, NORMAN L. *Introduction to Psychology*. Boston: Houghton Mifflin Company, 1962.

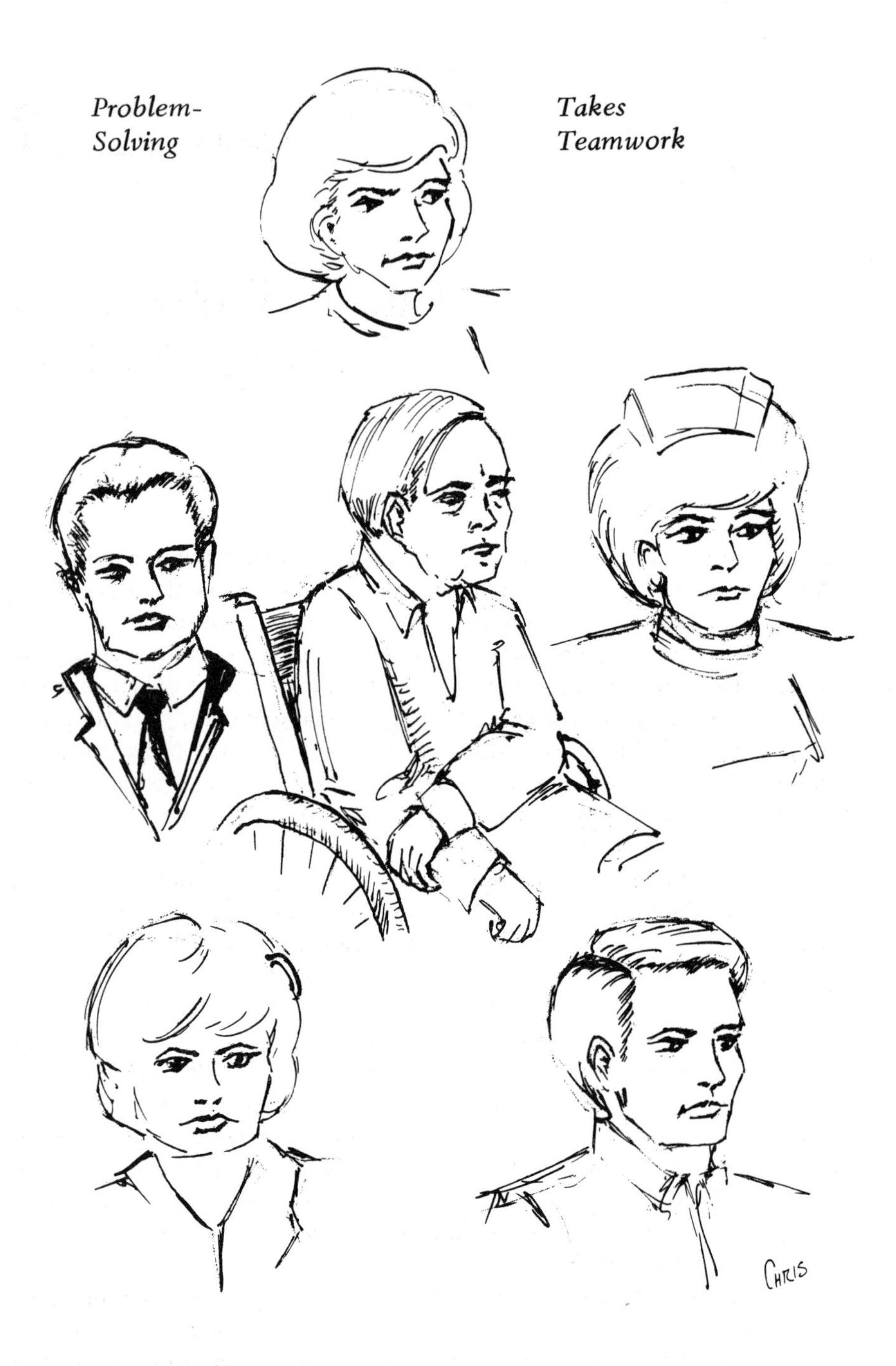
Problem-Solving
Takes Teamwork
CHRIS

Chapter 2

Patient Problems vs. Nursing Problems

The word "need" is a very "in" word in nursing today but like so many words in the English language it does not mean the same thing to everyone who uses it. Countless times teachers have said to students, "What are your patient's needs?" and the student has answered, "He needs a bath" or "A glass of juice" or "Companionship." Then teachers say, "Those are your nursing actions. Which needs are you trying to meet by them?" Whereupon, the student (sometimes the instructor also) thinks "what's the difference?" Because of this distress and confusion, we will present the ways in which this word "need" may be used and establish how it will be used in this book and why.

To the psychologist the word usually means a *feeling* of *necessity* to remove, allay, or correct conditions which are perceived as disruptions or deficiencies of self and of surroundings. In other words, it is a term used to convey the concept of *feeling* or *experiencing* a lack. To other psychologists and to many who serve in health and social occupations the word "need" represents those basic requirements of the body and psyche which the human being requires for health and survival. These are such things as food, oxygen, love, self-esteem, and communication with others. Lastly, it may be used to mean those items or actions which fulfill the requirement. It is often used this way in everyday conversation: "I need to go to the store," "I need to take a bath," "I need to fix dinner." In nursing, we say "the patient needs an enema," or "I.V.," or "more information."

As you can see all of these meanings are usable. The important thing is not to let the variety of meanings confuse and cloud the main issue and render the word useless for communication purposes. No matter how many meanings a word may have, it is still usable if the individuals agree on the meaning it will have for them.

In this book the word "need" will be used to represent the basic requirements of the body and psyche. In this connotation we have found it to be a valuable and useful word in nursing. The first definition is scientific and perhaps the most pristine use of the word but we have not found it practicable. The third meaning, while most common and certainly very usable, often leads to hasty conclusions about the action to be taken. Particularly for the beginner it tends to put the focus on the nurse's actions rather than on the patient.

An understanding of such psychological concepts as needs, desires, goals, motivation, will, conflict, and choice are vital to the nurse. The reader is urged to study these.

PHYSICAL AND PSYCHOSOCIAL NEEDS

There are certain tangible and intangible items (needs, requirements, essentials, necessities) which the human being must have in satisfactory amounts in order to attain and maintain physical and psychological homeostasis (equilibrium, balance). It is these upon which the nurse focuses when she encounters a patient situation. Her objective is to determine if the patient is experiencing an overload, deficiency, or is in danger of one or the other.

Maslow's categories may be translated into a suggested list of needs related to patients as follows: physiologic needs, safety needs, the need to belong, the need for recognition, esteem and affection, the need to create, the need for knowledge and comprehension and aesthetic needs (order, harmony, beauty).[1] His theory is that these categories encompass all of man's fundamental requirements and that they emerge in the order listed. Because the nurse practitioner must be as specific as possible in identifying the patient need in jeopardy, it is helpful to describe these categories in more detail.

Categories of Needs	*Description*
MASLOW	AUTHORS
1. Physiologic needs.	Comfort.
	Activity (rest and exercise). Correct body alignment and mechanical function.

[1]Abraham H. Maslow, *Motivation and Personality* (New York: Harper & Row, Publishers, 1954).

	Oxygen (includes circulation as well as respiration). Nutrients (protein, fat, carbohydrates, vitamins, and minerals). Elimination of wastes. Fluid and electrolyte balance. Regulatory function (hormone balance). Sensory and motor function.
2. Safety needs.	Freedom from threat of injury—mechanical, chemical, thermal, bacteriological, psychological, social, economic.
3. Need to belong.	Security, love, affection. Companionship. Productive relationship with others. Means of communication.
4. Need for recognition, esteem, and affection.	Self-concept. Self-identity (includes sex identity). Self-esteem, self-worth. Recognition. Awareness of individuality. Dignity. Respect.
5. Need to create.	Expression of self. Feelings of usefulness. Need to be productive, to contribute.
6. Need to know and understand.	Need for knowledge, understanding, comprehension. Need to control matters concerning self. Need to master self and environment.
7. Aesthetic needs.	Order. Harmony. Beauty. Truth. Privacy. A pleasing environment. Spiritual goals.

Abdellah and Associates identified twenty-one common nursing problems.[2] Needs of patients inferred from these nursing problems include:

1. Physical comfort.
2. Optimal activity.
3. Safety (mechanical, chemical, thermal, bacteriological).
4. Correct body alignment and satisfactory body mechanics.
5. Oxygen.
6. Nutrients.
7. Elimination of waste products.
8. Fluid and electrolyte balance.
9. Regulatory function.
10. Sensory and motor function.
11. Expression of feelings and reactions.
12. Effective means of communicating.
13. Productive relationships with others.
14. Achievement of spiritual goals.
15. Awareness of self as an individual.

These basic requirements (needs) are present regardless of age, sex, race, location, economic status, religious or political belief. They are necessary in health as well as during illness. They are essential whether the illness is physical, mental, or both; whether it is short-term or long-term; whether it is a major illness or a minor surgery. They are essential because of the physical and psychosocial nature of the human being. They are just as essential to you as they are to your patient. The difference is that *you* are able to meet your needs while the patient may require some assistance.

For the beginning student, an important point that should be gleaned from this discussion is: *You know more about the patient than you think you do.* Much of what you know about yourself is true also of your patient. While each person is unique and has a myriad of individual differences, he also has many characteristics in common with his fellowman. We would dare to say that the commonalities outweigh the differences.

OPTIMAL SATISFACTION OF NEEDS

People not only have a need for such things as oxygen, food, safety, and love, but they require certain amounts and kinds of each. Definite minimum and maximum amounts have been identified for some needs, for others we have only a general idea. As an example, while fluid and

[2]Faye G. Abdellah, et al., *Patient-Centered Approaches to Nursing* (New York: The Macmillan Company, 1961).

caloric needs are quite specific, it is difficult to say how much love one needs. The amount and kinds of items which meet the need often depend on age, weight, body surface, and circumstances. The nurse must be able to determine when needs are not satisfactorily fulfilled.

A number of factors influence these basic needs of man, causing a deprivation or an overload. It is important for the nurse to know what these factors are, what needs will most likely be affected by each factor, and how each need is most likely to be affected by the factors, that is, whether the factor will most likely produce deprivation or overload.

This knowledge will *guide* her when she begins her assessment. It will help her to know what needs to examine when she encounters a patient situation. For instance, when the nurse encounters a patient who is a six-year-old girl three days after an appendectomy, she will expect different needs to be apparent than when she encounters a forty-eight-year-old man one day after a severe myocardial infarct.

FACTORS WHICH INFLUENCE NEEDS

These are as follows:

Age and sex.
Type, location, and extent of pathology.
Levels of health or illness.
Type, extent, duration, and effectiveness of the therapy.
Available supply of the items needed to fulfill the need.
Physical, intellectual, emotional, and financial capability.
Education.

The factors are interrelated and affect one another. Age will affect intellectual capability. Pathology may influence physical and/or emotional capability. Education may affect financial status. Environment may influence the pathology one acquires.

The following are only a few influencing factors: Age and sex often have an influence on certain needs. These may affect the amount of calories and specific nutrients needed, the amount of fluids necessary, or the amount of rest required. For instance, caloric requirements are less in childhood than in adulthood; adolescent and adult males usually require a lighter caloric intake than females of the same age; rest needs are high in childhood, decreasing with adulthood, and increasing again in senescence.

In the example of type, location, and extent of pathology, a physical illness is more likely to affect physical needs, whereas a mental illness will probably affect psychosocial needs. They each have an effect on the other, however. Infectious processes may cause different deficits than neoplastic or degenerative processes.

Location of the pathology or injury makes a great deal of difference. Obviously more needs as well as different needs will be affected if the pathology is in the brain as compared to the little finger. If the pathology is extensive it usually causes greater deficiencies in more areas.

Pathology located in the bowel will interfere with elimination. A fracture of the femur will deprive the patient of one of the most important means of exploring his environment, thereby obtaining information about himself and his surroundings. If the pathology is located in the brain all areas of need are likely to be affected. The more vital the organ affected, the more serious the repercussions.

The influence of the extent of pathology on needs demonstrated by patients almost speaks for itself. To emphasize the point, consider how many more need areas would be affected if the patient has cancer of the lungs metastasizing to the neck and bones, than if there is an early cancerous lesion on the cervix of the uterus.

Level of health or illness means somewhat the same thing. It is simply whether you prefer to look at how healthy you are or how sick you are. Even when we are considered "healthy" we never have a perfect level of wellness. Once some pathology is evident one is commonly referred to as "sick" or "ill" or "injured." One, however, does retain some level of health or "wellness." They are two sides of the same coin. The person then either "gets better," his level of wellness increases, or he "gets worse," his level of wellness decreases.

The point at which the patient is in the course of health or illness will affect his needs. Following are some examples.

The first and second day after admission to the hospital for croup (acute spasmodic laryngitis), a three-year-old's physical needs for oxygen, rest, regulatory function, and fluids will be significantly affected. In addition, he will be extremely frightened and struggling for breath. He will be separated from his family and familiar surroundings. These factors increase his need for security and love.

Six days later, when the clinical manifestations (the signs and symptoms) have abated, the needs which will assume importance will most likely be for food, exercise, safety, recognition, companionship, and identity.

FAILURES IN PHYSICAL AND PSYCHOSOCIAL DEVELOPMENT

When needs are not met in early life, interference with physical and/or psychosocial development may result. The person may then have a health problem as he grows older. Many times the person will adapt in some way especially if the need deprivation has not been severe. If so, he may never bring the problem to the medical/nursing team. Sometimes as he gets older he may become more aware that he has a prob-

times as he gets older he may become more aware that he has a problem. Perhaps someone at school or work will help to recognize that something is wrong and encourage him to seek help. Failure to recognize inadequate physical development occurs but more often it is the lack of psychosocial development that is not noted. This is partly due to the fact that it is often not as obvious as a missing or underdeveloped body part and partly because our culture has tended to be less understanding of psychosocial problems. Another reason is that we do not have as many tools for detecting failures in psychological growth and development as we do for detecting failures in physical growth and development. In recent years more emphasis has been placed on mental health and more people are seeking help.

We are making a special point of this because many people who come under the care of the physician and nurse for treatment of some physical pathology have failures in psychosocial development. Due to the stress of illness or hospitalization their compensatory mechanisms may not be adequate and the developmental failure may become more evident. This does not mean they become psychotic but only that they are not as psychologically or emotionally healthy as someone else. At these times their mistrust, shame, doubt, guilt, inferiority role, anxiety, etc., may become more evident. This in itself can constitute a patient problem and, in turn, a nursing problem.

Present nursing students and recent graduates are more fortunate than their predecessors. This area of knowledge necessary to give better care has been included in their education. Lack of formal education, however, in the psychosocial development of man need not be an obstacle to any nurse since there are many excellent texts available to all who wish to enrich their background. This additional knowledge will provide more acute recognition of the widely accepted developmental tasks of each age. With this added ability, the nurse will more clearly understand why a patient may be having more than the obvious physical problems.

Once having increased her store of theoretical knowledge of man's development in relationship to family and society, it then follows that the ability to transfer this knowledge is necessary. Just as the nurse uses scientific principals to improve her physical care of the patient, so the principals of psychosocial needs may serve to more fully cope with these problems. Once again the use of the steps in problem-solving are employed. One note of caution: the nurse should recognize her own limitation in this field if the problem appears too complex, and be wise enough to seek further help. Support for the patient in this situation will aid in reaching the level of wellness desired.

PATIENT PROBLEM vs. PATIENT BEHAVIOR

As previously stated a need is a basic requirement. It is considered basic and required because unless it is fulfilled, that is, met to a certain specificed degree, physical and psychological balance will be disturbed. It is this physical and psychological balance that we call health. If a person's needs are over-fulfilled or under-fulfilled, the balance is disturbed. This disturbance is referred to as a patient problem.

A patient problem is the disturbance in need balance, e.g., ischemia (lack of oxygen and nutrients to a body part). The disturbance in turn causes some physiological and/or emotional behavior.

A patient behavior is any sign, symptom, act, or response made by the body as a whole or by a part of the body or the actions and responses made by the total person, e.g., cyanosis, pain. The behavior may be very evident or quite subtle. If we can observe the response it is called a sign or overt behavior. If it cannot be observed by one of the five senses but must be elicited by examination of and for communication with the patient, it may be called a symptom or covert behavior. Anyone may note the behavior—the patient, his family, an aide, an x-ray technician, the nurse, the physician. While anyone may note it, the members of the health team are expected to note it, but every member of the health team is not expected to do so with the same amount of skill. Naturally the physician is expected to have the greatest skill but cannot be with all the patients at all times.

Therefore, when constant observation is deemed necessary the doctor places the patient under the care of the nursing team which is expected to have skill in observation of patient behavior. The nursing team is made up of various kinds of nursing personnel: the aide, the orderly, the licensed vocational or practical nurse, and the registered nurse. Each of these team members has different educational preparation and varied experiences. Their observational skills will be proportional to their preparation and experience.

Sometimes the patient notes the behavior and realizes that it indicates a disturbance. Sometimes he can define the disturbance. Most of the time he simply deals with the behavior. For example, he may note that he is constipated and recognize that this is disturbance of his need for adequate bowel elimination. He may then take a laxative. He may never know exactly what the actual disturbance was but if his action is successful he is satisfied.

While the person is under the care of a physician and the nursing team, he may also note his own behavior. He can then tell the physician and the nurse what his symptoms are. The patient is always the best source of information about himself. However, many times he is too ill or too distracted by the total situation to be aware of any behavior except the most obvious and most distressing. Rarely does he have the knowledge to define specifically what problem the behavior indicates. This is a function for the doctor and the nurse.

The patient problem usually falls into one of the following categories:

1. *Deficiency*—e.g., loss of muscle tone, ischemia, deficient cardiac output, loss of blood, inability to inspire or expire, loss of electrolytes, loss of identity, loss of role.

In this category we find the lack or loss of a function (inability to digest, inability to move, inability to trust) or a deficiency of a needed item (food, oxygen, fluids, love).

2. *Overload*—e.g., excessive heat production, hyperemia, increased blood volume, increased demand for oxygen, overprotection.

In this group we find problems of input above the normal safety range and also problems of demand beyond the person's ability to compensate (either physiologically or psychologically).

3. *Danger*—e.g., danger of injury, dehydration, loss of body image.

A real danger can be said to constitute a patient problem. Recognizing and defining significant danger so that an actual problem may be prevented is most important.

Although we have classified problems in one category or another it is not always quite this clear-cut. In many instances deficit and overload occur together. For example, a lack of rest often occurs in combination with an excess of exercise or increased demands for rest; cardiac output may be deficient if there is an increased demand for circulating blood. Often there is an overload of work placed on an organ. If the demand continues and the organ cannot adjust to the demand there will appear to be a deficit. Deficiencies in their turn can cause an increase in demand and this results in the problem of overload of work. An example of this is a deficit of blood volume due to hemorrhage. When this occurs the heart has to work harder to meet body demands.

It is not the purpose of this book to teach you the different kinds of patient problems, the behavior they produce, and the circumstances in which they occur. You learn that as a part of your nursing education, continued study, and experience. The following illustrations may aid you in understanding what is meant by a *patient problem*:

Patient Need	*Patient Behavior*	*Patient Problem*
Fluid balance for adult: 2000-3000 c.c. per 24 hours.	Thirst. Dry skin. Oliguria Constipation.	Deficiency of water for all body cells. Intake 1000 c.c. below requirements.

Knowledge and an understanding of events concerning himself.	Fails to carry out requests: appears anxious and frightened.	Lack of information about himself and his situation.
Knowlege. Information	Confused. Actions are inappropriate to situation.	Unable to correctly perceive himself, others, and/or his environment.
Elimination of waste products.	Distended bladder. Discomfort.	Inability to void.

NURSING PROBLEMS

The nursing problem is the question which must be answered in order to assist the patient to solve his problem. One could say, instead of problem, nursing goals, aims, or objectives. Nursing Problems fall into three main categories or questions:

1. How can we maintain the need balance?
2. How can we correct the disturbance?
3. How can we relieve or minimize the distressing behavior?

To be more specific they can be phrased in any of the following ways depending on the situation:

How can we	(maintain (promote (facilitate (provide (increase (supply of)	(that which meets the patient's (needs (and (behavior?
How can we	(remove	(the cause of disturbance?
How can we	(accept, allow the expression of	(the behavior? (
How can we	(prevent (alleviate (eliminate	(the problem? ((
How can we	(teach	(the patient and/or his family (to do one or several of the (above?

This appears very simple. In one way it is; in another way it is not. It is simple inasmuch as we are really saying, "the patient's problem is that something is wrong and the nurse's problem is to help him set things right again." It is not so simple when you consider that the nurse must identify as specifically as possible what the disturbance (problem) is and then state specifically what problem she must solve in order to correct the disturbance. It is the difference between saying,

> "My patient has a disturbance. How can I correct the disturbance?"

and saying,

> "My patient has a disturbance in heat regulation. He is producing more heat than he is eliminating."
> "How can I facilitate his elimination of heat? How can I reduce his production of heat?

This also illustrates the difference between simply noting the patient's physical behavior and identifying his problem. We do not minimize the importance of observing behavior for more is expected of the nurse than that. She must know what the behavior means when viewed in relation to other behaviors and circumstances in a given situation. When she can do that we say that she is making a nursing diagnosis. The act of diagnosis or identification of the problem is explored and illustrated in Chapter 3.

The doctor is the only one who may determine (diagnose) the pathological cause of the problem, name it, and prescribe a course of action to treat the pathology. He is the one who can say, "this patient has a fever (behavior), his problem is a disturbance in heat regulation, and the cause of the problem is a pneumococcal infection in the lungs." This last phrase constitutes a medical diagnosis.

The nurse can say, "the patient has a fever; the problem is he is producing more heat than he is eliminating." This can be said to constitute a nursing diagnosis. When the doctor has made his diagnosis, the nurse is expected to know what kind of behavior this disease is likely to produce and to be on the lookout for it. When the doctor has not yet made a diagnosis the nurse is expected to note all behavior and report and record it to aid the doctor to reach a diagnosis. In either case, the nurse should be able to identify the physiological or psychological disturbance.

THE NURSE AND IDENTIFICATION OF PATIENT PROBLEMS

You may think that if the physician notes the behavior or is told of it, if he knows what the problem is *and* knows what the pathological cause of the problem is, why does the nurse have to know? Is she not doing a job someone else has already done and perhaps done better? Is it not enough for her to observe and report behavior and do what the doctor tells her? No, it is not, not if nurses are to be more than robots or automatons; not if nursing acts are to be intelligent acts; not

*Patient Behavior**	*The Cause may be Pathological, Developmental, or Circumstantial***	*Physical and Psycho-Social Patient Problem*	*Medical/Nursing Problem*
Cough.	Pneumonia.	Overload of secretions in the lungs and bronchial tree.	How can we reduce the accumulation of secretions?
Cyanosis of toes.	Thomboangiitis obliterans.	Ischemia and Hypoxia—a lack of blood supply to the part and consequently a lack of O_2 to the tissue.	How can we increase the blood supply to the foot? How can we minimize tissue demands for O_2?
Hemoptysis.	Tuberculosis of the lungs.	Blood Accumulation in lungs.	How can we decrease bleeding in the lungs?
Plantar flexion of the foot (footdrop).	Lack of exercise. Poor nutrition.	Loss of muscle tone.	How can we prevent loss of muscle tone? How can we support the foot in a functional position? How can we increase muscle tone?
Tissue breakdown over sacral area. (decubitus)	Prolonged pressure on bony prominences.	Local ischemia and hypoxia.	How can we increase blood supply to sacral area?
Unaware of environmental hazards.	Age 1 year. Anesthesia.	Danger of physical injury.	How can we protect patient from injury?

Generalized skin discomfort.	Bedrest. Unable to bathe.	Accumulation of oils, perspiration, and bacteria on skin.	How can we remove the oil, bacteria, and perspiration from skin?
Nausea and vomiting. Semi-conscious.	Anesthesia.	Danger of aspirating vomitus into lungs.	How can we prevent aspiration?
Hypotension.	Cardiac decompensation or failure.	Inability to maintain cardiac output; disproportion between cardiac output and body demands.	How can we increase cardiac output? How can we decrease demand for cardiac output?
	or	or	or
	Surgery or anesthesia affecting the sympathetic nervous system.	Peripheral vasodilatation: Vascular bed is larger than available blood volume.	How can we reduce the size of the vascular bed?
	or	or	or
	Gastric hemorrhage. Ruptured aortic aneurysm.	Loss of blood volume.	How can we restore the blood volume? How can we stop blood loss?

*The response made by the body, psyche or both, to the causing factor or factors.
**The causes given here represent one example of many possible causes.

*Patient Behavior**	*The Cause may be Pathological, Developmental, or Circumstantial***	*Physical and Psycho-Social Patient Problem*	*Medical/Nursing Problem*
Diarrhea.	Gastroenteritis.	Failure to reabsorb water in large intestine; deficiency of water supply for all body cells; danger of dehydration and electrolyte imbalance.	How can we increase reabsorption of water in large intestine? How can we prevent dehydration and electrolyte imbalance?
Dyspnea.	Pulmonary Emphysema and Fibrosis.	Inability to exchange oxygen and carbon dioxide in the lungs.	How can we increase the exchange of O_2 and CO_2? How can we decrease the body's demands for O_2?
	or	or	or
	Myasthenia Gravis.	Inability to use muscles of respiration.	How can we facilitate the act of respiration?
Expresses marked skepticism. Expresses doubts about care. Very demanding. Makes requests in a dogmatic, arrogant manner.	Deprivation of parental love in childhood. Deprivation of safe environmental years. Physical needs unmet as an infant.	Is unable to trust.	How can we decrease his doubts about the quality of his care? How can we help the patient develop some degree of trust in her relations with the health team and possibly with others.

Sometimes expresses ambivalence towards his family and the staff. Often belittles himself. Looks and takes little interest in his appearance.	Loss of a love object—either real or imagined.	Feels worthless.	How can we facilitate the process of grief and mourning?
Feelings or expressions of self-deprecation. Expresses both love and hate for family and close friends. Hostile to himself. Says he wishes he were dead or that he had never been born.	Manic-depressive psychosis. Schizophrenia. Involutional melancholia. Reactive depression.	Lacks a sense of self-worth. Feels worthless. Danger of self-injury or suicide.	How can we help the patient to develop feelings of self-worth? How can we prevent hostility toward himself?

*The response made by the body, psyche or both, to the causing factor or factors.
**The causes given here represent one example of many possible causes.

if nursing is to be a science as well as an art. Here are some concrete reasons.

First of all, although the doctor does recognize the problem and its cause and writes orders for therapeutic action, he does not indicate exactly what every problem is and designate which order is for each behavior, problem, and cause. Sometimes he does but not always. He may write:

Aspirin grs. X for temp. over 102°

but he may also write a number of orders such as

Demerol 100 mg. I.M. q. 4h. p.r.n.
Compazine 5 mg. I.M. q. 4h. p.r.n.
Aspirin grs. X oral q. 3 to 4h. p.r.n.
Coronary regime
Diet as tolerated

Now the nurse must implement these orders. She must decide when to employ them and when not to employ them. She can do so safely and intelligently only if she too knows what the problems are for which each is intended.

Secondly, there are problems for which most doctors do not write orders. Problems in the danger category are a good example. The nurse is expected to know what dangers are present in a given situation and take action to prevent them. For example, the problem of decubiti is always present in bedridden patients who cannot move about well. Danger of injury is often present for young patients and patients whose level of consciousness or awareness is decreased. The doctor rarely writes orders to cope with these problems.

Psychological or emotional problems are often left for the nurse to identify and deal with, especially in the general hospital or at home. Other problems are created by the circumstances rather than the pathology. An example is respiratory obstruction following inhalation anesthesia. The nurse is expected to identify these problems and take action. Often there are no doctor's orders nor is there time to get them. If the unconscious patient's tongue is obstructing his airway the nurse is expected to identify this and correct it.

The following includes some examples of situations in which there is both pathological cause for the physiological and/or psychological problem and some examples of situations in which the cause is not pathological but is developmental or circumstantial. You will note that the final column illustrates the medical/nursing problem. The heading was decided upon to emphasize the team work of the medical and nursing teams. The nurse is rarely involved in patient care unless the doctor is first involved. Therefore, it really becomes a joint problem. For some problems the doctor has the exclusive right to choose the course of action. He may carry out the action himself, as in the case of surgery, or he may delegate the performance of the action to the nurse, for example, administration of medications. For other problems, the nurse has the right to plan care. She may then carry out the action herself or delegate it to another member on the nursing team who has the required skill. Many times they plan care together. Regardless of who plans the course of action and carries it out, both the medical team and the nursing team are obligated to keep each other informed. Finally, it is the nurse team leader who formulates a plan for the nursing team which incorporates both the doctor's choices of action and the nurse's choices of action.

It is important that the nurse identify the problem (disturbances), not just the behavior. However, sometimes one cannot identify the problem and sometimes nothing can be done about the problem. In these cases, all that the nurse can do is reduce the distressing behavior. Consider, for example, pain arising from a surgical incision in the abdomen. The disturbance in the sensory nerve endings in the skin, subcutaneous tissue and muscle is evident but you can do nothing about it. The body itself in time will correct the disturbance. In the meantime, you can minimize the pain (behavior) by administering medication ordered by the doctor and through such independent nursing actions such as placing the patient in certain positions or providing support at incision site when the patient moves.

In another case, your patient may exhibit the symptom pain in the wrist and knee joints due to arthritis. The problem may be identified as inflammation and accumulation of fluid in the joints. In this situation the medical/nursing team may be able to attack the problem by providing rest to reduce the inflammation and by applying heat to increase circulation and reduce the accumulation of fluid. In addition, an analgesic may be administered at safe intervals. In this situation an attempt is being made to do something to alleviate both the disturbance and the behavior.

Looking at another patient situation in which the problem is more covert, Mr. Taft has had an amputation of his leg below the knee. The wound has healed, there are no complications and a prosthesis has been provided. Mr. Taft, however, does not wear the prosthesis. Instead, he finds other means of locomotion. Many times the problem is identified as "patient will not wear the prosthesis" and the nursing problem as "how can we get Mr. Taft to wear his artificial limb?" Some critical thinking will reveal that this is really his behavior, not his problem. Further assessment must be done. Perhaps then it will be discovered that Mr. Taft fears that he will fall or that he fears failure or lacks confidence, or that he has not accepted his loss. When the real problem has been identified the nursing problem can be recognized and plans formulated to solve the patient's problem. When the problem is solved, the behavior will disappear.

Before concluding, some mention should be made of other kinds of nursing problems. They are those which pertain to the nurse's own function, those which are her own problems of accomplishing her assignment or carrying out the activities of her position. They may be stated this way:

```
          (plan          (
          (organize      (
How can I (work          (the whole assignment or
          (direct        (the parts of a
          (evaluate      (specific activity?
          (replan        (
```

These are challenging nursing problems and the ability to solve them is important to nursing practice. They are, however, essentially the same problems that are found in any kind of job which involves planning, directing, and organizing. Books have been written on the application of problem-solving methods to job organization and management. You are urged to seek them out and study what they have to say and apply the suggestions in your daily activities. Believing that a book was needed to demonstrate the application of the methods of problem-finding and solving to problems related to patients' needs, the text of this book has been directed to this task only.

PRIORITY OF NEEDS AND PROBLEMS

Maslow and others support the theory that there is a hierarchy of needs, that is, that they can be arranged in order of rank. Maslow contends that man will meet his most basic needs first, and not until these are met will other needs emerge and ask to be met. He states that man will first seek to meet his physiological needs (oxygen, food, fluids, etc.). When these needs are met, then his need for safety will emerge and demand to be met and so on through each category. A knowledge and understanding of these concepts is most valuable to the nurse.

That man's physiological needs must be met before his needs to belong, create, know, and understand, etc., certainly has implications for nursing. It is important, however, to understand that the physiological needs demand to be met in preference to other needs only when the deprivation is life-threatening. It does not mean that a man will eat his lunch in preference to talking with his wife who can only visit at that moment. This man's need for food is not truly unfulfilled. On the other hand, there are situations in which the patient's physiological needs do demand to be met over all other needs. If the patient's respiratory tract is obstructed and his need for oxygen is not adequately met, this takes priority over his safety and all other needs. In this case, a tracheostomy might be performed without insuring bacteriological safety (that is, performed without sterile technique) and certainly no one would delay action in order to meet the need to know what is taking place or to meet the needs of recognition, esteem, and affection.

This is priorities of needs in its most basic sense. But priorities also occur in another sense. They may occur among specifics within a category. For instance, one physiological need may take preference over another. There are times when the need for food is greater than the need for rest. In other words, the deprivation of food is greater than the deprivation of rest. This can also happen among all the categories. While not totally deprived of any need, a person may be more deprived of one need than another need.

There are times when two needs ask to be met at the same time. As an example, consider a situation in which one has a need for food, rest, and recognition. If the latter need is great enough, a student may forego both food and rest to put in extra hours studying in order to achieve a better grade, or a man may work extra hours to achieve a promotion.

As a nurse, you will most likely be assigned to care for a number of patients. Each of these patients will have needs and problems that create nursing problems. If one of your patients has three problems at the same time or three of your patients have one problem at the same time then you will have three nursing problems simultaneously. Now the nurse's situation becomes: Which problem do I solve first? Which second? How can I work on all of them in the time allotted to me?

You will have to solve both kinds of nursing problems. To do this you must constantly decide which problems have priority. If you think about it for a minute you will immediately realize that not all problems are of equal importance or urgency.

Suppose, for example, that you assess a patient's needs and identify the following problems:

1. Lack of peristalsis resulting in abdominal distention and pain.
2. His skin is unclean due to inability to bathe.
3. He has a disturbance in heat regulation—temperature orally is 100.2°.

You cannot work on all of these problems at the same time. You decide which one takes priority. Since the lack of peristalsis is creating the most distressing behavior, you solve that one first. Let's say that there is a doctor's order for a Harris Flush. You give this and achieve some relief. Then you bathe the patient and make him comfortable in a clean bed. The increased temperature may represent a slight problem but it is most likely a compensatory reaction of the body to injury (the surgery) and may be relieved somewhat by the flush and bath and then by rest and administration of fluids.

Sometimes a number of very important patient problems will occur at the same time. How many of them the nursing team can solve will depend on the number of problems and number of nursing personnel available. The most vivid example of this is often seen in the emergency room when a large accident or community disaster has occurred.

Through your basic educational program and through continued experience and education you develop your ability to make wise judgments in these situations.

SUMMARY

Physical and psychological needs are the essentials which the human being must have in satisfactory amounts in order to attain and maintain homeostasis. A number of factors, such as location of pathology and effectiveness of therapy, can influence needs. The nurse uses this knowledge to identify unsatisfied or over-satisfied needs. It is also desirable to predict areas in which the need might not be satisfied. Preventive action could then be taken.

When needs are not met some changes usually take place. Whether the change is minor and local or whether it involves the total person depends on the need affected and the degree of deprivation or overload. These observable changes or behavior alert the patient and/or the health team members involved and provide clues to the patient's problems.

The patient's problem is the disturbance in his need balance. It may be a deficiency, that is, "a loss or lack of" or "an inability to. . . ." It may be an overload, that is, "an excess or increase of . . ." or "an increased demand for. . . ."

The nursing problem is the question the nurse or nursing team must answer in order to assist the patient to solve her problem. It is the goal, aim, or objective of the nursing team.

It is important for the nurse to recognize patient needs and problems and to establish the nursing goals in relationship to them. There are numerous daily problems which the patient faces during his illness with which the nurse can help him cope. Sometimes the nurse helps the patient by carrying out a prescription from the doctor. There are numerous other instances in which the nurse assists the patient to solve her problems by independent nursing action.

An important nursing function is to decide which needs have priority in a given situation. The amount of time and personnel available will influence the number of patient's needs that a nursing team can meet at one given time.

Suggested Reading

ABDELLAH, FAYE G. "Methods of Identifying Covert Aspects of Nursing Problems," *Nursing Research* (1957), 6:4.

ABDELLAH, FAYE. *Patient-Centered Approaches to Nursing*. New York: The Macmillan Co., 1961.

BELAND, IRENE L. *Clinical Nursing: Pathophysiological and Psychosocial Approaches*. New York: The Macmillan Co., 1965.

ERICKSON, ERIK. *Childhood and Society*. New York: Norton Publishing Co., 1950.

HOFLING, CHARLES K.; LEININGER, MADELEINE M.; and BREGG, ELIZABETH A. *Basic Psychiatric Concepts In Nursing*. 2nd ed. Philadelphia: J. B. Lippincott Co., 1967.

VAN SANT, GENE E. "Patients' Problems Are Not Always Obvious," *American Journal of Nursing*, 65:59, 1962.

Problem-Solving Means

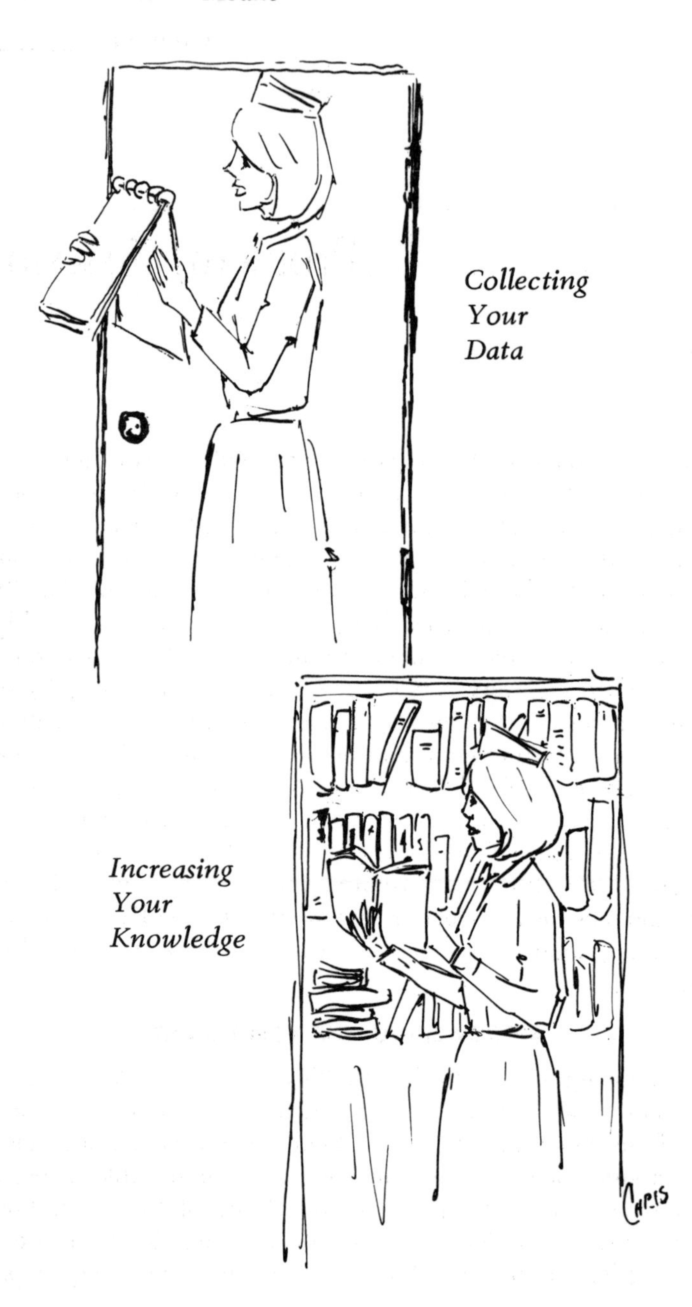

Chapter 3

Problem Assessment

Each time you care for a patient you will be assessing his needs. You will assess, then reassess, and assess again. It is an ever-constant part of nursing. No patient situation is static; rather it is ever-changing. Different needs are affected by each change in the patient's condition, by the time of day, and by the various circumstances of the situation. Each patient has each need listed in Chapter 2, and it is possible for a patient to have a problem relating to any one of them. To consciously assess each need for every patient, however, would be a lengthy process. You must, therefore, decide which needs require your attention first. This gives you a starting point and helps you to make the most judicious use of the time available. This is where you recall and apply your knowledge. As you approach the assessment of your patient, recall what you know about anatomy, physiology, pathology, therapy, and the needs of his age group. Recall the facts from psychology, sociology, microbiology, physics, and chemistry which relate to this particular situation. Then focus your attention on the needs which you think will most likely be affected.

APPROACHING THE ASSESSMENT

The following is an attempt to illustrate what takes place in the nurse's mind as she approaches the patient situation. To describe a true picture of the nurse in action is difficult. In the actual situation many mental activities occur at the same time. It is impossible to portray all of this on paper and still preserve the clarity of the illustration. The nurse's mind is never dealing with only one step in the process even when caring for one patient. When she is caring for a group of patients, the situation is compounded. While in the *act* of bathing one patient, the nurse may be *formulating a plan* to increase his range of motion, and almost simultaneously she may be assessing the respiratory status of the patient in the next bed. With experience the nurse's mind is able to move from one step to another and back again according to the various situations she encounters.

The following situation is simplified in order to demonstrate what takes place in the nurse's mind related to assessment.

Imagine that it is 3 p.m. and you have just arrived on duty. You are assigned to care for four patients. The following information is given to you in report:

1. Christopher Smith, age 16, returned from surgery at 1:30 today. Scleral buckling O.D. Bedrest. Not to turn for 24 hours. Liquid diet. Still drowsy. Has not voided.
2. Mrs. Andrew, 40 years old, 3 days postcholecystectomy. Has been ambulated twice today. Had medication for pain once. Taking a full liquid diet with no difficulty.
3. Mr. Arthur, age 76, bronchial pneumonia. Admitted 8 days ago. Up and about in his room ad lib. Receiving a soft diet. No elevation of temperature. Seems comfortable.
4. Mrs. Long, age 38, admitted 3 days ago with diagnosis of reactive depression. Ate a little bit of breakfast but refused lunch. Doesn't want to bathe or dress. Says "Why bother." Becomes very irritable when nursing staff tries to encourage her to do these things.

Now consider each of the above patients and list the needs most likely to be affected by their individual situation.

1. Christopher Smith, age 16 years. Day of surgery. Scleral buckling O.D. Most likely to be affected in this situation are his needs for:
   a. perception of his environment
   b. comfort
   c. safety
   d. fluids
   e. urinary elimination
   f. control and mastery of his situation
   g. rest
   h. love and affection (sense of belonging)
2. Mrs. Andrew, age 40 years. 3 days postcholecystectomy. Most likely to be affected in this situation are her needs for:
   a. bowel elimination
   b. exercise
   c. nutrition
   d. mastery of self and environment
3. Mr. Arthur, age 76. 8th day in hospitail. Bronchial pneumonia. Most likely to be affected in this situation are his needs for:
   a. optimal activity (rest and exercise)
   b. oxygen

c. recognition; self-esteem
d. usefulness; productivity
e. psychological comfort (freedom from fear)

4. Mrs. Long, age 38 years. 3rd day at hospital. Reactive depression. Most likely to be affected in this situation are her needs for:
   a. self-worth, self-esteem
   b. hygiene
   c. nutrition
   d. optimal activity (rest and exercise)
   e. acceptance
   f. recognition
   g. communication
   h. meaningful relationships

USE OF KNOWLEDGE IN FOCUSING ASSESSMENT

The nurse is able to postulate that these are needs most likely to be affected because of knowledge she possesses about each situation. She knows what needs are affected by age, sex, pathology, and therapy. From the above examples consider Christopher. The following is an example of what would go on in the nurse's mind before making an assessment. (Of course, she would not state everything this formally. One tends to recall knowledge in a more overall way.)

Recall that Christopher's needs are most likely to be:

a. perception
b. comfort
c. safety
d. fluids
e. urinary elimination
f. control and mastery of his situation
g. rest
h. love and affection

Knowledge	*Implication*
The retina is that part of the optic nerve which spreads out over the posterior inner aspect of the eyeball. The retinal nerve endings transmit visual impulses to the brain where they are interpreted. A retinal detachment is a separation of the retina from the choroid. This causes a loss of vision.	Chris will have lost some of his ability to perceive himself and his environment.
A scleral buckling is a surgical procedure which aims to affix the choroid and retina and promote reattachment. Approximation must be maintained if success is to be achieved. Approximation is maintained by keeping the eye at rest. The eye rests by keeping the whole body quiet. Often the doctor will require the patient to stay flat in bed to help attain reattachment.	This means there is a danger of discomfort and lack of exercise. Rest needs will be increased. This may cause some venous stasis in the lower extremities, back, and buttocks.

Knowledge	*Implication*
Eye movements are almost constant in the act of seeing. Both eyes move simultaneously, therefore, both eyes will probably be covered after surgery.	Chris will be unable to obtain visual perception of his environment.
General anesthesia depresses the central nervous system. Sometimes this results in inhibition of impulses to the musculature of the urinary tract.	The patient may be unable to void for 24-48 hours.
General anesthesia tends to increase mucus secretions in the respiratory tract.	Patient is in danger of respiratory tract infection.
Perception is influenced by one's physical and emotional state, size, past experiences, values, interests, and current needs. Perception influences behavior whether or not the perception is correct.	Chris may misplace articles, knock things over, misjudge distances, etc. This may influence his safety. He may also respond inappropriately to others. He may be frightened.
Man needs satisfying relationships with others to maintain mental health.	Chris may be lonely. His need for companionship may be increased.
One's sense of person, time, and place is affected by prolonged sensory deprivation.	Chris may become confused or disoriented with both his eyes covered.
A change in body image threatens the self-concept. Threats to self-concept produce anxiety.	His need for self-esteem may be affected. He may feel anxious.
Some people must maintain control of themselves and their situation in order to feel physical and psychological safety. The dependence on others caused by illness constitutes a loss of control.	Chris' need for mastery of his situation may be affected.
The skin continually collects oil and debris. Accumulation of these on the skin causes discomfort to many people. Lying in bed in more or less one position makes it difficult to bathe and may increase perspiration.	Chris' needs for hygiene and comfort will be affected.
Perspiration, venous stasis, anxiety, unfamiliar environment, pain, etc., stimulate the C.N.S.	His ability to sleep and/or rest may be affected.
Fluid intake was probably curtailed for 8-12 hours (prior to anesthesia and during surgery).	His need for fluids may not be met.

This example is not all inclusive but it serves to illustrate the base of knowledge from which the nurse proceeds and how she applies it. It enables her to focus her attention on specific needs. Without this knowledge it would be necessary to rely on the patient or someone else to identify what dangers or problems are present. The nurse's primary objective, however, is to *anticipate* and *prevent* problems. If she has to wait for the problem to occur before taking action she would give very poor nursing care indeed.

To focus implies that you bring your object into view as clearly as possible. The act of focusing prepares your mind for the closer examination in which you observe and communicate with your patient and use all other sources of information available. You will then become aware of things you could not perceive from a distance. You may discover some of the needs that you suspected were not really evident and that some needs were unexpectedly revealed.

Perhaps when you visit Christopher you see that his mother and brother are present. Talking with them reveals that he is one of six children and that the family takes turns staying with him so that he is rarely alone. His high school friends also plan to visit. Knowing this you may be less concerned about his need for love, affection, and companionship. Safety (physical and psychological) would probably be assured. You might, however, be more concerned about his need for rest.

You focus a scene with a camera in order to bring your object into perspective and to eliminate distractions on the periphery. In nursing, it is also desirable to focus on the patient situation and try to bring your object (his needs) into the most advantageous perspective possible before assessing (taking a picture of the situation). Do not focus so rigidly that you create a "mind-set." This could cause you to overlook dangers or problems outside your focus. On the other hand, do not omit establishing some goals for your assessment. If you do, it may result in failure to recognize problems, and valuable time may be wasted.

SOURCES OF INFORMATION

In the nursing situation the best sources of information are:

1. The patient.
2. The patient's family and friends.
3. The chart.
4. Members of the nursing team.
5. Members of the health team.
6. Books, journals, and experts.
7. Yourself.

The Patient

No one knows more about his situation, his needs, and his problems than the patient himself. He may not be aware that he knows due to the lack of insight or lack of intellectual development. He may not be able to communicate information clearly due to lack of vocabulary or because of a speech impairment. He may not wish to impart information because he fears he will embarrass himself or others, or perhaps, because he wishes to protect his family's privacy. Nevertheless, the information, in large part, lies within the individual. Trust and rapport must be established between the patient and the nurse. Then, through the skillful use of interviewing techniques, the patient may be helped to recall and/or reveal information.

Reference is made not only to information about intimate, personal problems or even to the wide range of psychosocial needs and prob--lems that were listed earlier. It is often necessary to establish a relationship and search for information about physical problems. It may surprise the inexperienced practitioner how often a patient will *not* tell you he has pain, is hungry, does not like his room, is too hot or too cold, is nauseated, and so on. The nurse may be sensitive to such needs and create an atmosphere which helps the patient to feel free to discuss his needs. When the patient cannot or will not give you information, you must seek it from other sources.

Family and Friends

If they are available and if it is appropriate to ask information of them, family and close friends are an excellent source of information. When the patient is unable to speak for himself, as for example in the case of a child or an unconscious person, they are usually the major contributors.

These people are frequently neglected by the nurse as sources of information. This seems to be due partly to the fact that many nurses are not comfortable *talking with people* (as they are comfortable doing for people). They are not at ease with the patient and they are even less at ease with his visitors. They are inept at the art of conversation and the science of the interview, and thus they rationalize that they do not want to "meddle" in the personal affairs of their patients or do not wish to infringe on the family's visiting time. Rarely do we see a nurse intentionally make "rounds" during the height of the afternoon or evening visiting hours. Hence the family members or the friends appear and disappear from the patient's hospital life never asked to do anything except to take the patient home when therapy is completed. Those who have the most right to share in his life—or death— and probably have the greatest need to contribute are the most denied.

The patient and his family, of course, suffer the most from this neglect but the nurse loses too. How can the nurse truly know and experience this person apart from his family and friends? She cannot. After all, he has been Mr. Adams, patient, for a very small part of his life. He has been Mr. Adams—husband, father, brother, friend, business associate, employer, employee—for a much longer time. This is the person as he sees himself; the person as others see him. Some people never see themselves as a "patient." Seeing the patient as he sees himself enables the nurse to help him identify and solve his problems. By getting to know his family and friends, by talking with them, by obtaining information from them, the nurse is better able to see the PERSON who is the patient.

The Patient's Record

The patient's current record as well as previous records are sources of information. The "chart," as this record is called in hospitals, contains the medical history recorded by the doctor and the findings of his physical examination. There are "notes" written by the doctor and the nurses recording the therapy and treatments carried out and their observations of the patient's responses to his illness, therapy, and hospitalization. Many times, however, they record only physical responses, thereby giving only half a picture. The chart also contains the reports of diagnostic studies and the reports of other members of the health team such as the physical, occupational, and nuclear therapist.

A word of caution! The chart is a valuable and useful source of information but it should not be used to the exclusion of other sources. It never tells all.

Members of the Nursing Team

The nursing team may be made up of registered nurses, licensed vocational or practical nurses, technicians, aides, and orderlies. We have already pointed out the various kinds of education an R.N. may possess. In the hospital she holds such positions as staff nurse, head nurse, supervisor, director of nursing services or team leader, clinician, clinical expert, depending on the hospital's job classification format. The L.V.N. or L.P.N. (depending on whether you live in the Western or Eastern United States) usually has twelve months of education. All classes are taught by registered nurses giving elementary theory in anatomy, physiology, nursing, pharmacology, psychology, and microbiology.

The technician such as the surgical technician and psychiatric technician usually receive nine to twelve months of classes specifically oriented to the area of concentration. Aides and orderlies may have anywhere from six hours to six weeks of classes usually given by the employing institution or some agency in the community which prepares aides for several local hospitals. Some aides have had no specific classes and were prepared on the job by the "buddy" system. These people are not licensed.

The group of people on the team with you will have information to share about your patients. The value of the Team Conference is that it provides a definite time for sharing information and making plans for patient care.

Members of the Health Team

The nurse is only one member of the overall health team. The dietitian, physical therapist, inhalation therapist, psychologist, social worker, housekeeper, pharmacist, pathologist, and radiologist are some of the other health team members who serve the patient and his family.

Obviously if they are participating in the care of your patient they will have valuable information to share with you and will need to obtain information from you. The benefit the patient derives from the team's effort is usually only as great as the nurse's ability to facilitate communication between team members. To draw an analogy from our ever popular western movies, the doctor holds the reins and chooses the route but it is usually the nurse who keeps the wagon train together and all the parts cooperating. The doctor is the Wagon Master but the nurse rides Ramrod. Again, Team Conferences are a useful vehicle for the transmission of information.

Books, Journals and Experts

This source of information is indispensable to student and practitioner alike. As previously stated, one must have information to apply. To make an intelligent assessment the nurse must have knowledge of the needs that are of particular importance in the patient's situation, what constitutes a need deprivation, that is, what constitutes a problem, and what fulfills these needs. She must understand the scientific basis—the physiological, pathological, psychological, microbiological and sociological reasons—for the patient's physical and mental health problems. There has to be an understanding of the medical goals and plans and the scientific principles underlying the therapy instituted.

Much of this information is acquired during the years of formal education. Through reading and discussion, the student acquires knowledge and learns how to apply it. Experience, too, is a great school of education. Experience and study complement and reinforce each other.

There will always be gaps in our knowledge. Even the so-called "expert" does not know all. But we must endeavor to close these gaps as much as possible. New information is constantly being discovered and the practitioner must keep abreast of it. This can be done by keeping our own library up to date and by using the libraries available at local schools of nursing or at our place of employment. There are several excellent nursing publications available now that can be subscribed to and read. *The American Journal of Nursing* is the official magazine of the American Nurses Association. Also recommended are *Nursing Outlook, Nursing Forum, Nursing Research,* and *R.N. Magazine.*

Lectures and workshops are also excellent ways to enhance one's knowledge. The state and local divisions of the American Nurses Association usually sponsor a number of educational programs throughout the year. In some states the Board of Nurse Education and Nurse Registration holds annual or semi-annual programs on a statewide basis, and, of course, the colleges and universities offer not only workshops and lectures but many courses open to the practicing nurse.

Remember this: While one cannot know everything, one can know where to find needed information. When you know "where to look it up," you are smarter than you realize.

Yourself

Last but not least, there is you and the store of knowledge you build up within yourself. If you do a good job, you will be, in large part, your own source of knowledge. This is most important. As you assist others to solve problems you are often the missing link in the chain of facts. You must put all the data together and add to it those missing pieces of information from your particular field of expertise. After all, is this not why the patient has sought your help? You serve him when you bring to him your knowledge. In a way, these last two categories merge. Much of what is in the books and the journals and the minds of experts and researchers must ultimately be transferred to your own mind. In the course of the nurse's busy day she can rarely run off to the library, and even the number of times she can ask information of another is limited. The nurse must have some knowledge in her head and be able to use it.

Consider Mr. Ronald and the nursing diagnosis: danger of forma--tion of a decubitus. The nurse might arrive at this diagnosis by making the following assessment.

Information from the Patient

1. Appears (while lying in bed) to be tall and thin.
2. Grey hair.
3. Facial expression appears sad.
4. Unable to move right arm or leg.
5. Full range of motion in left arm and leg.
6. Speaks with no difficulty.
7. Says that before his "stroke" he was leading an active retirement life. Had formerly been an electrical engineer. He particularly enjoyed bridge, reading, and gardening.
8. Has a wife, who is well, two sons and three daughters—all married. Three live nearby and he enjoys his family and grandchildren.
9. His symptoms occurred suddenly a week ago. Since then he has been hospitalized. His only previous hospitalization was as a child.
10. Says he gets up in a wheelchair three times a day for about an hour.
11. When he is in bed he says he lies primarily on his back as it is difficult for him to turn himself.
12. He eats fairly well but has little appetite and "hospital" food doesn't taste like food at home.
13. The aide bathes him each morning and he gets a back rub at night.
14. The physical therapist gives him exercises twice each day but he "doesn't see any good coming of it."
15. Redness appears over coccyx after only 10-15 minutes of lying in bed.

From Chart

1. Sixth hospital day.
2. Diagnosis: cerebral vascular accident, left side.
3. Age 69.
4. Doctor's orders: Multi-vitamins i o.d.
   Ferrosequels i B.I.D.
   Chloral hydrate grs. VII h.s. p.r.n.
   Up in wheelchair at least T.I.D.
   Encourage activity.
   Physical therapy B.I.D.
   Regular diet.

From Nursing Team

1. Aide says that she and the orderly get Mr. R. up in the wheelchair after his bath in the morning and again about 1 or 2 p.m. Mr. R. is lifted from the bed to the chair. The evening aide confirms that they do likewise once on the evening shift.
2. Aide says she bathes Mr. R. in the a.m. He helps a little with his left hand but being right-handed he is not able to do much.
3. Evening aide says she rubs his back at least twice and turns him on his side at least once. The night nurse turns him once or twice.
4. Aides and nurses say there is no evidence of skin breakdown.

Family

His wife and son say the family visits regularly but hesitate to attend Mr. R. as they do not believe they should. They say that both he and they are very discouraged.

From Health Team

1. Physical therapy record shows that Mr. R. receives passive exercises to his right arm and leg B.I.D. Muscle tone is being maintained.
2. Doctor's progress notes say "condition improving slowly."

(This appears on paper like a great deal of information. In actuality it was gathered in a relatively short period of time.) Now recall that the problem identified was danger of a decubitus forming. (He, of course, has numerous other problems but we are taking this one as an example.) How do you know that is the problem? Even with this fairly thorough assessment the problem does not naturally flow from it. There are more facts which must be supplied. These come from your store of knowledge.

1. The skin is supplied with blood vessels which bring oxygen and nutrients to maintain cell life.
2. Pressure reduces the lumen of the blood vessels and hence reduces the amount of blood which can pass through them.
3. The weight of the body against the mattress produces pressure particularly over bony prominences.
4. Constant pressure may deplete the blood supply and cause injury to the skin.
5. The body gives off heat. Rubber and plastic (with which mattresses are frequently covered) are not good conductors of heat.

When you put these facts with the ones you have gathered you should be able to deduce the problem. In a subsequent chapter an examination of the process of putting facts together and arriving at a conclusion will be discussed. The main point here is that *you* must be able to supply scientific information pertinent to your goal. *You* form the link between the patient and his problem. This is a large part of the service for which he is paying you. If he had the knowledge and skills with which to find his own problems and had the knowledge and skills with which to solve them, he would not seek nursing service (unless, of course, he were too weak physically to use his knowledge and skill, but this would be a small percentage of all patients). It also reemphasizes the point that the more knowledge the nurse has and the better she is able to use it (knowledge is worth nothing if you don't know how to use it), the greater will be her skill in problem-finding and problem-solving. From this point it should follow that the more education a nurse has (obtained through *both* study and experience), the better able she will be prepared to problem-find and problem-solve.

METHODS OF OBTAINING INFORMATION

There are two major methods by which information is imparted and received: verbal communication and nonverbal communication.

The Communication of Information

The current literature is replete with material on this subject. Only a brief discussion will be presented here, the aim being merely to give communication its place in the overall scheme of problem-solving.

The word "commune" comes from the old French word *communer*, meaning "to share." The act of communication is that by which two or more people share information. It implies both giving and receiving. It may involve words, verbal communication, or it may be done by other means, in which case it is known as nonverbal communication. There are many techniques for using each method and one can develop skill in the use of these. The larger the number of techniques one is skilled in using, the greater will be the quantity and quality of information gathered.

Since success in problem-finding and problem-solving is largely dependent on the information one can gather and recall, it follows that the more skillful the practitioner is in communicating, the more skillful he will be in problem-solving.

Influencing Factors

Before considering the methods by which we communicate it is important to consider the three elements involved: the sender, the receiver, and the message. The personality, culture, education, mannerisms, voice, vocabulary, skill and intention of the parties attempting to communicate will influence the results. The content of the message, the time at which it is received, and the place in which it is received will affect its reception.

Nonverbal Communication

Messages may be sent without words by one's behavior, i.e., by one's responses to a stimulus; by gestures, signs and symbols, pictures, and by sounds other than words. Art and music are certainly means by which people communicate their thoughts, impressions, and feelings. When the audience applauds, laughs or cheers, they may be communicating their approval.

A person's behavior reveals much. He may laugh, cry, scream, be silent. The way a woman keeps house, the manner in which a man conducts business, the games a child plays, all tell something about the individual.

The body also responds to stimuli in certain ways, thereby communicating messages to us. Pain, fever, cough, cyanosis are ways the body has of telling us that something is happening.

The method by which messages are "picked up" is *observation*. To observe means to look at, to inspect, to examine, to scrutinize, to review. The senses transmit these impressions to the brain for analysis and evaluation.

Observation Through Sensory Perception

It is primarily through the eyes that most nonverbal communication is received. We *see* how a person acts. We *see* the events which stimulate, and we *see* the conditions of his environment. This information gives us clues to his intellectual, emotional, and social capabilities.

Science has in recent years provided mankind with many devices which extend his natural eyesight. Such instruments as opera and field glasses, telescopes, microscopes, and cardioscopes are examples. Television is being used more and more in medicine and nursing, both as a method of teaching and as a means of monitoring patient care. The x-ray machine and fluoroscope allow the doctor to see inside the human body. New developments in photography are permitting events to be recorded and viewed at later dates.

The nurse uses her eyesight to perceive such things as skin color, character of respirations, color and amount of drainage, swelling, and facial expressions which indicate comfort or discomfort.

Much delightful information comes to us through the sense of smell —freshly baked bread, coffee brewing, and the scent of pine trees in the mountains or orange blossoms in the springtime. This sense also receives messages which could mean danger such as something burning.

The sense of taste can also bring pleasant or unpleasant messages. A chicken dinner, apple pie, and champagne may bring pleasing sensations, whereas the taste of soured milk or spoiled food may warn us to be careful.

The sense of smell is particularly important in nursing where it can detect a musty odor beneath a cast, a foul odor from dainage, an unpleasant odor to breath or skin, or the smell of something burning in a patient's room.

The body receives a number of sensations through receptors in the skin: heat, cold, dryness, moisture, pressure, and pain. The nurse uses her sense of "touch" or "feel" to detect indications of physical change in her patients. Through the use of this sense it can be determined if his skin is hot or cold, dry or moist. Size, shape, and texture can also be determined. Local swelling (edema) and enlarged organs can be felt (palpitated) by the nurse and doctor. The nurse can use her hands and other objects to elicit skin sensations in the patient. The thermometer and the potentiometer are instruments which extend the sense of touch.

Emotion and psychic response may also be communicated and detected through the sense of touch. Recall how much a handshake may have told you about another, the many messages you have sent and received from loved ones by a touch or a kiss, the times you have been encouraged by a mere "pat" on the arm. On the other hand, if someone throws a rock at you or kicks you in the shins, you will surely detect anger or hostility. The patient and the nurse also learn much about each other through the way they touch each other.

Words are the sounds which we most often *hear*. There are, however, many sounds other than words which we observe without ears. Each minute of the day the sounds of our environment are transmitted to us. When we are conscious of them and have learned to interpret them we can gain valuable information. Thunder tells us a storm is approaching, the bells at a railroad crossing that a train is near, "folk-rock" music that the kids are home.

The nurse's ears must be ever alert to sounds from her patients and from their environment. Breath sounds, heart sounds, and bowel sounds can be heard with the aid of a stethoscope. Noisy respirations, choking, gasping, sobbing, screaming, laughing—all these can be observed with the sense of hearing.

Verbal Communication

We speak or write when we wish to send messages with words. Both of these require a command of the language used: an adequate vocabulary, both of general words and of specific terminology (if such exists), an ability to spell, and an ability to structure sentences correctly. If the message is written, the communicator must be able to produce the letters and symbols involved in a clear and legible manner.

Verbal communications are "picked up" by *reading or listening.* As with speaking and writing there are requisitions to be fulfilled if the methods are to "work." Above it was stated that to hear is not necessarily to listen. Listening implies attention to what is being said and a conscious effort to understand the message. People do not always say what they mean or mean what they say. To hear and to understand without bias or prejudice is essential to the process of problem-finding and problem-solving.

In conclusion, some of the people with whom you will communicate may lack skill in any or all of the methods of verbal and nonverbal communication. Many will have physical and emotional conditions that impede communications. Your skill will make up the differences. In other instances, the people whom you serve and with whom you work will have assets which far exceed your own. In such a case you must recognize your limitations with humility. It is not unusual for a beginning student to find that *she* is being "assessed" by her patient. The student may find that even in simple conversation the patient is both initiator and sustainer. She need not be upset by this. Fortunately, patients are warm, wonderful people, just someone's mother, father, brother, sister, aunt, or uncle. Let them help you to learn how to communicate. And while you stand there, quietly allowing them to "talk" to you with their voice, their hands, their eyes, you will have learned the most valuable lesson in communication: the importance of conveying the message that you accept the other person and are both willing and able to listen to him.

Exercise:

Discuss the following situation with a group and determine what response would encourage the patient to express his problem and which would hinder communication.

You are in the process of answering Mr. Dale's light and as you pass the room next to his you catch a glimpse of the patient's bed in that room. The spread and the blanket are almost completely on the floor and you make a quick mental note to return there as quickly as possible. You pass a second time on your return to the utility room to fulfill Mr. Dale's request, again noticing the next room where an elderly man patient in the bed is raised up on both elbows with a faintly worried expression on his face. Within the next few minutes you are able to return to this patient. You find him perched precariously on the edge of the bed with an even more worried expression. You enter the room and approach the patient. What is the patient's need?

Would you say something like the following, and if so, what kind of response might you expect?

1. Is anything wrong?
2. May I help?
3. What's the trouble?
4. Why are your covers almost off the bed?
5. Get back in the bed before you fall.
6. You look uncomfortable. I would like to help, if I may.
7. Why are your covers almost on the floor?

Would you DO any of the following, and if so, what might the response be?

1. Introduce yourself.
2. Excuse yourself quickly (because you are a stranger) and go find out who is in charge of this patient.
3. Say nothing and simply start straightening the bed.

Consider the responses: "Get back in bed before you fall." Most likely there will be a tone in your voice with this kind of remark that may not be too friendly. Can you envision the kind of reaction you might possibly get from the patient? Do you think it will be easy for him to tell you what his problem is? Will he feel you are scolding him? Is there a chance that he might respond with an angry, resentful expression?

You might say: "May I help?" Depending on the nature of the problem you might get a negative response. It is possible that the patient might be too embarrassed to tell you what his problem is. He may feel he needs to provide you with a suggestion as to what you may do to help and yet not know what is best to do. If he was embarrassed or uncertain, this might add an additional problem for you along with whatever appears on the surface to be wrong. However, he may give you just the answer you need to go ahead and assist him. He may also be very angry about the entire problem and wonder why the male nurse who had been assigned to him had not returned instead of you.

Or, you introduce yourself "I'm Miss Matthews, a nursing student from the Center City College." If the patient is obviously not very comfortable at the moment, how do you think he will respond to your rather formal even though courteous approach? Will he be apt to introduce himself in return? Will he be happy that, at least, you came into the room? Will he be made more uncomfortable by thinking that since *you* appear to be in command *he* should try to quickly adjust to meet the situation in a polite and courteous manner even though he appears very uncomfortable? Will he resent your ability to be up and about when he is not so able? Will he just ignore the introduction and explain his problem?

Or the question, "Is anything wrong?" Just what kind of a response might you get from that question. Will he think you are just asking a silly question when by all indications something is wrong? Will he be glad you came in and, at least, asked?

Or would a combination of two or three of the questions be more in order? For example, you might say "Is there anything I can do here to make you more comfortable? You seemed so anxious as I passed by just now; I would like to help you if I may." This gentleman might be very frightened and the tone in your voice might dispel fear. He might be able to tell immediately that you know something is wrong and he need only explain and you'll try to help.

Before interpreting the information you have gathered, and drawing a conclusion from it, you must stop to critically examine the data. This may take only a moment or it may take hours or weeks, depending on quantity and complexity of the information, your experience with similar matters, and the urgency of the situation. The accuracy of your conclusion (your nursing diagnosis) is of vital importance to your patient. His physical and mental health depend on it. Since your conclusion is based on the information collected it is essential that the information be valuable, accurate, and sufficient in quantity. Ask yourself:

1. Are the facts correct?
2. Do I have all the facts I need?
3. Were the sources of information reliable?
4. Is the information I have relevant to the problem or situation?
5. Do I have enough information to draw a conclusion?
6. Have I been as objective as possible in gathering information?
7. Have I considered the possibility that bias or prejudice (on my own part or on the part of others) may have obscured the facts?
8. Am I clear about the meaning of what has been communicated to me?
9. Was the meaning of the words used clear to all?

This examination phase can be considered part of the assessment. As mentioned in Chapter 2, it is often done simultaneously. You acquire a piece of information, examine its usefulness, and keep or discard it accordingly. Experience helps you to know what kind of information you need. Whether you look at it as part of the assessment phase or the beginning of interpretation, or as the bridge between, does not matter. The important thing is that the examination of the data is not neglected. Careful and intelligent examination should reveal whether or not you have a sufficient amount of pertinent information. It may be that the only conclusion you can draw is that you do not have enough facts upon which to base a judgment. It seems from our experience that this happens more frequently than most people would like to admit. The "rush to judgment" or the "jumping to conclusions" is a most common and human characteristic. It is often an undesirable trait. In nursing, as in medicine, law, psychiatry and ministry, it may be dangerous if not fatal. When a person chooses an occupation in which he says to the public "I will serve you by guarding your health, your rights or your soul" and "by helping you make judgments and decisions," he also chooses a serious responsibility. He must be well prepared to undertake the responsibilities and functions implied and conscientious enough to always do his best. If you have to make decisions for others then you must strive to make the best possible ones. Consider the following situation.

The aide brings a message to the nurse. "Mr. Thurman wants something for pain." The nurse gathers a few more facts.

1. The patient is 46 years old.
2. Diagnosis: ruptured appendix.

3. 2nd day postoperative appendectomy.
4. Received medication for pain 5 hours ago.
5. May have Demerol 100 mg. I.M. q 4 hr. p.r.n.
6. There is a tranquilizer order but he has not had any.
7. There are no other influencing drugs ordered.

She then concludes that Mr. Thurman's problem is incisional pain caused by the surgery and proceeds to attempt to alleviate or eliminate the problem by administering the Demerol. The nurse enters the patient's room and says, "Mr. Thurman, I have an injection for you." The patient obligingly prepares to receive the injection and the nurse administers it. Now the following conversation ensues:

Mr. T.: I sure am miserable.

Nurse: That's understandable, but the injection I just gave you should take away most of the pain caused by your surgery.

Mr. T.: Oh, I haven't much pain there. I'm just so uncomfortable in this position. That bottle (pointing to the I.V.) was started four hours ago and the nurse told me to lie still until it finished. Now the aide says I have to get another bottle. I told her I'm just too miserable and can't stand any more. She said she would tell you.

Nurse: It's true that you should keep your arm relatively still but you can turn and move about a bit. The I.V. is running well and the needle is taped securely.

At this point the nurse assists Mr. T. to exercise his legs, turns him on his side and rubs his back.

Mr. T.: "Oh, that's wonderful. Now, I wish I hadn't taken that injection. It makes me so sleepy and a little nauseated and my wife will be here in about a half hour. I didn't realize that's what it was. I thought it was penicillin or something.

Now review and look for steps in the problem-solving process the nurse skipped.

1. The nurse encountered a problem situation.
2. She assessed the situation.
3. She interpreted the facts.
4. Drew a conclusion.
5. Plan of action was then selected and carried out.

Obviously the nurse did not make a thorough assessment nor did she carefully examine the facts gathered. Both are important. You could say that if your assessment was well done you would not need to examine it. But how do you know if the information you have gathered is significant, pertinent, complete, and objective unless you examine it? This does not mean that in every instance you have to list all your information and sit down and think it all over in an elaborate or lengthy process. Sometimes, particularly with psychosocial problems, this may be necessary. In many of the frequently encountered situations in nursing the urgency of the situation does not permit it and the relative simplicity of the problem does not require that the examination be lengthy or detailed. Nevertheless, one must take time to examine and do it conscientiously. At the very least mentally run through those questions listed under "Examination of the Data." Do I have all the facts? Am I making assumptions? Have I clarified the words used? and so forth.

In the situation above the nurse should have attempted to clarify the meaning of the aide's statement before doing anything else. This could have been done by asking the aide "Did Mr. T. actually say the word 'pain'?" If so, "did he say what kind of pain he meant and where?" If the aide could not answer these questions, the nurse could then go to the patient's room and verify the situation through direct questioning.

Suppose the aide answered, "Well, he didn't exactly say 'pain' but he said he felt miserable and couldn't stand any more." Then, even if the nurse went directly to the chart for further information and gathered the facts as listed above she should have stopped for a moment again to ask herself, "Do I have all the possible facts that tell me what the problem is?" "Are there any other possible causes for discomfort?" The three or four seconds it takes to do this are usually well worth the time spent. If the nurse had gone to the patient for information, the time spent preparing the medication would have been saved. In addition she would have correctly identified the problem. Nurses often say there isn't time for all this examination, that it is all right in theory but not in reality. However, when the problems are incorrectly identified and incorrect plans are carried out then more problems are usually created. In the long run more time is lost than saved.

The above example illustrates the necessity of assuring yourself that your information is sufficient in quantity and valuable in quality. Further elaboration is necessary to establish the correct meaning of the messages sent and received and to control bias and prejudice.

Clarifying Messages

Suppose your data contains such pieces of information as "patient has not voided for several hours" or "there is quite a bit of drainage on the dressing." The words "'several" and "quite a bit" are relative terms. They do not mean the same thing to everyone. There are many such words: large, small, long, short, fat, thin, high, low. When attempting to communicate measurement, more precise terms can and should be used.

Unfortunately, terms of measurement are not the only words in our language which cause confusion. Individuals attach a wide variety of meanings to words and language symbols. Even people with similar educational and cultural backgrounds and similar work activities find that word meanings vary widely. To test this, ask a classmate to define a word he or she would commonly use. Your authors found this to be ever so true as they collaborated in writing this book. If the nurse is to obtain correct and useful information it is necessary to clarify the words used in our communications with patients and their families and with fellow workers. This latter included the doctor. Unfortunately, communication between doctors and nurses is frequently a one-way street with no attempt made by either party to clarify the message received. This often happens when people see each other in an authority-subordinate relationship. When the patient sees the nurse as an authority figure he may not ask for clarification of her message. The nurse can help everyone involved, including herself, to send and receive clearer messages by asking, "Did I understand you correctly?" "Did you mean. . . .?" or "Did you understand me?" "Tell me what you heard me say." This device could also be used more frequently in teacher-student communications.

You must keep reminding yourself that your information must be the best it is possible for you to acquire so that your diagnosis will be accurate. Then you will carefully choose those words which have limited meaning in order to say exactly what you intend to say. You will find yourself observing and listening more attentively and critically to the other person to determine if he understands you.

Attaining Objectivity

Webster's New World Dictionary defines *Objective* as an adjective meaning "concerned with the realities of the thing dealt with rather than the thoughts of the artist, writer, speaker, etc.; without bias or prejudice." *Subjective* is defined as an adjective meaning "of or resulting from the feelings of the person thinking rather than the attributes of the object thought of."

You will easily recognize that it is difficult for human beings to achieve objectivity at all times. Because of this, the nurse must continually examine the information gathered for the influence of emotion, prejudice, bias, or personal inclination. You have all watched detective shows and can recall instances where a number of witnesses described the same event quite differently. We tend to see what we are accustomed to seeing or what we want to see. We look at people and events out of our own frame of reference, that is, out of our own background and experience. Many things influence our perception—our family background, culture, education, experience. This is why, in a previous chapter, you were urged to read and study about how man perceives and what influences him.

As has been said before, you will acquire much of the information from the patient, his family and friends, and from other members of the health team. The very fact that there are so many individuals involved increases the possibility of subjective information. In addition to this, many patient problems are subjective in nature: pain, itching, weakness, fear, anxiety, distrust, boredom. Add to this the inevitability of your own subjective analysis and the almost certain possibility that you will have a very short time in which to make your analysis, and you can see the dangers involved. *Be on your guard. Be ever ready to allow for these subjectivities.*

It is possible to improve one's objectivity through constant effort and experience. It often helps to compare your observations with those of others, thereby disclosing your own subjective tendencies.

Exercise: Try testing your objectivity by assembling several people to describe a person or event and then explore together the description.

SUMMARY

Assessment is the most vital part of the process. The nurse must obtain a *sufficient* amount of *pertinent* information in order to diagnose the patient's nursing needs. Unless the patient's need is correctly ascertained it cannot be met.

When the nurse encounters a patient situation she recalls knowledge from the various physical and behavioral sciences which can help her postulate what needs might be affected by the pathology and circumstances. This enables her to focus her attention on specific need areas as the assessment begins. It is wise to have certain objectives in mind before starting to make an assessment, nevertheless remain aware of other possibilities.

Utilize as many sources as possible to determine patient needs. Become as skillful as possible in techniques of verbal and nonverbal communication.

Carefully examine and validate all information.

Suggested Reading

Bermosk, Loretta Sue and Mordan, Mary Jane, *Interviewing In Nursing.* New York: The Macmillan Company, 1964.

Hays, Joyce C. and Larson, Kenneth, *Interacting With Patients.* New York: The Macmillan Company, 1963.

Kron, Thora, *Communications in Nursing.* Philadelphia: W. B. Saunders Co., 1967.

Peplau, Hildegard, "Talking With Patients." *American Journal of Nursing,* 60:964-66, July, 1960.

Travebee, Joyce, *Interpersonal Aspects of Nursing.* Philadelphia: F. A. Davis Co., 1966.

Problem-Solving
Means
Checking Your Choices
For The
Best Solution

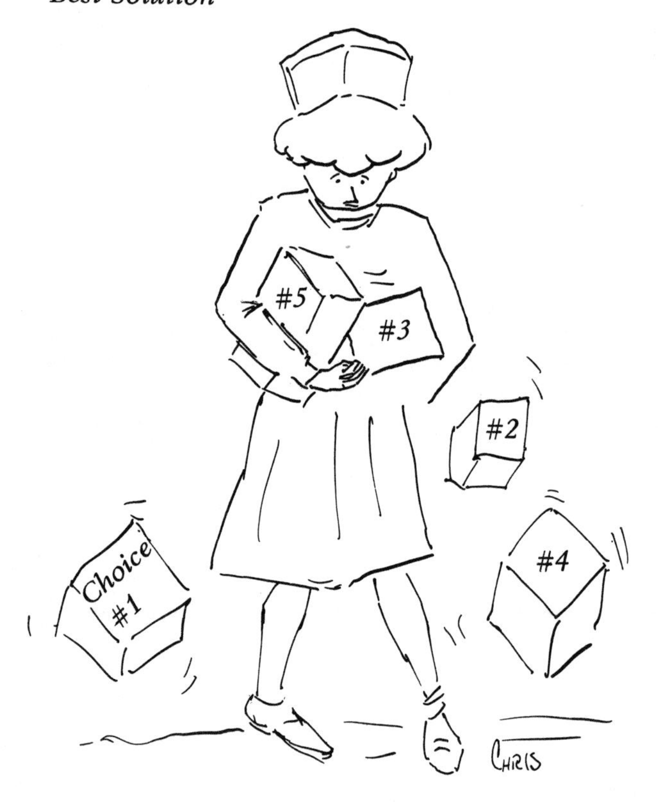

Chapter 4

Problem Statement

When you have made every effort and feel sure that your information is correct and complete, begin your interpretation. If assessment has been thorough and information has been validated, interpretation is usually not difficult. It can safely be said that failure to recognize the problem or to identify the correct problem is due in most instances to an inadequate assessment and a careless examination of the data. This does not in any way minimize the importance of interpretation. As you well know, the most thorough and accurate data can be misinterpreted.

In order to correctly interpret the information gathered, the nurse must

1. Have knowledge.
2. Be able to utilize that knowledge.
3. Be able to recognize the meaning of the relationships between the facts.

PROBLEM IDENTIFICATION

Once the nursing history and physical examination have been completed, that is, the assessment has been made and the information examined, you are ready to decide what the problem is. You do this by making relationships between the facts, recognizing the meaning of these relationships and concluding that a certain definite need disturbance is present or imminent. Prince and Durand call this "recognition of a pattern."[1] The way in which you do this in your mind is very difficult to describe. It involves a comprehension of the facts, a defi-

[1]Mary Durand and Rosemary Prince, "Nursing Diagnosis: Process and Decision," *Nursing Forum*, Vol. V, No. 4, 1966, pp. 50-64.

nition of their meaning, an ability to see how the various facts relate to one another and to what conclusions these relationships point. You learn to do this through study and experience.

Perhaps the best way to explore this process is to take a situation which you might come upon in your personal life. You get into your car in the morning to go to school or work and the car doesn't start. You have encountered the situation.

The first thing you must know are your car's needs and the kinds of disturbances that can occur. You know that your car needs such things as gas, water, and perhaps antifreeze. All of its parts must be there and able to function. What disturbances can occur? It can have too much or too little of a need item or one of its parts may be unable to function.

With this knowledge at your disposal you make an assessment. You focus on the needs and try to find out which are not met. You acquire the following information:

1. All the parts are there—nothing has been stolen.
2. There is gas in the tank.
3. Radio plays.
4. No horn.
5. No lights.
6. No ignition response.

You add the following information from your knowledge:

1. The battery supplies electrical power for ignition, lights, horn, and possibly radio.
2. Gas is fuel which burns on ignition and sets up compression and energy.

By now you have already decided upon the problem: The battery is "dead." In reality, this whole process would probably have taken no more than two or three minutes. *How* did you arrive at your conclusion? Most likely you have had this problem before or been present when someone else had such a problem. From past experience or through instruction you recognize the pattern. You were able to see the relationship between the facts gathered and the knowledge you had.

No response to turning the key to the ignition, no horn, no lights, plus knowledge that the battery supplies electrical power for ignition equals loss of battery power.

This is a simple situation, the facts are few, and the conclusion relatively obvious. The illustration shows that the *process* by which you arrived at this conclusion is the *same process* used in identifying patient problems. Simple, obvious problems also occur in nursing and may be as quickly identified. Other situations are more complex, the assessment produces numerous facts, a large amount of scientific knowledge is added by the nurse assessor, and the conclusions are anything but obvious.

Recall the example of Christopher. This example showed why the nurse must have the necessary knowledge in order to have some ideas about the needs which might be affected in a given situation and to speculate on what problems might be present or apt to occur. In Mr. Ronald's case, the nurse added the information collected from the patient and various other sources to her own store of knowledge. The two are mentally combined and a conclusion drawn (problem identification and nursing diagnosis). It is difficult to show mental processes on paper but this gives you the idea. Durand and Prince give a number of excellent illustrations of this.

Once you have arrived at a conclusion, the natural thing to do is to put it into words, at least to phrase it in your own mind. For example, you might say to yourself, "Looks as if Mrs. Kelton's problem is her inability to void and my problem is to find a way to help her empty the bladder." This takes place as such a natural part of your thought process that often you do not even realize that you have stated the problem. If you are the only one who needs to know what the problem is, this mental statement is enough. If, however, it is necessary to involve others—the patient or members of the nursing team—in formulating plans and carrying out actions to prevent or alleviate the problem, then the patient's problem and the nursing problem (or problems) must be verbalized by oral or written means.

THE PATIENT AND STATEMENT OF THE PROBLEM

You may think that the patient knows what his problem is since he is the one who has it. This is not always so. Sometimes he knows he has a problem but does not know specifically what it is. Many times he is only aware of some physical or psychological discomfort. For example, he may be aware that he is uncomfortable but not aware that his specific problem is bladder distention. Sometimes the patient knows what his health problem is but does not know what general problems he must face in order to solve his *health* problem. Finally, there are times when the person does not even know that he has a problem. Many people have incorrect posture (body alignment), unhealthy skin, decaying teeth, limitations of eyesight or hearing, inadequate nourishment, disturbances in elimination, lack of confidence, or loss of identity, (to mention only a few), and do not know it.

It should be remembered that the patient is a key person on the team. In most instances it is imperative that he understand what his problem is and accept its validity. In the case of a child or an unconscious or confused adult, it is usually necessary that those responsible for the patient (usually the family) understand and accept the problem. Only then will he and/or they be willing to participate in reaching a solution by: (1) suggesting ways of alleviating the problem; (2) definite acts which contribute to relief of the problem; or (3) allowing the health team to do those things for him or to him which work toward a solution.

Nursing and other health occupations endeavor to do that for the patient which he is unable to do for himself. We always want to maintain or promote as much independence as possible and not take away the right of the individual. Keep in mind that the person retains the right to accept or reject help and the right to select the kind of assistance he wishes. On the other hand, it is our obligation to do everything possible to help the patient understand what his health problem is and what means are available to solve it. Only then can he freely choose to take action and only then can he choose wisely.

THE NURSING TEAM AND PROBLEM STATEMENT

For the nursing team this is a two-fold job. The team must understand what the patient's problem is and what the nursing problem is. It is just as important to state the nursing problem as it is to state the patient's problem. The team must know what its objective (aim, goal) is. By this we mean that all members of the team involved in the care of a given patient are consciously aware of the specific goals which are to be attained. The team cannot be expected to make a unified effort toward the nursing problem unless they know what it is.

Specific Statement

The beginner usually makes the mistake of not stating the patient's problem or behavior specifically. Consider the following:

1. Lack of oral hygiene.
2. Loss of muscle tone.
3. Impaired range of motion.
4. Pain.
5. Danger of injury.
6. Danger of infection.
7. Lack of fluid balance.
8. Lack of knowledge.
9. Anxiety.

These are examples of patient problems but they are so general it would be difficult to plan nursing care to resolve them. Impaired range of motion could mean anything from inability to raise the arm to inability to move all the joints in the body. In order to develop a plan to solve or alleviate the problem, it must be stated more specifically and reflect the individuality of the patient's situation.

Now take those same problems and restate them in more specific terms. Assume that the nurse has thoroughly and correctly assessed the needs of Mrs. Leigh, a 52-year-old person with rheumatoid arthritis. She evaluates the information gathered and states the problem as follows:

1. Mouth dry, tongue coated, lips cracked.
2. Loss of muscle strength and tone in arms and legs.
3. Unable to flex knee and wrist joints.
4. Inflammation and swelling of knee and wrist joints, pain in all joints.
5. Danger of falling when getting in and out of bed.
6. Danger of respiratory infection.
7. Fluid intake 500-600 c.c. below need.
8. Lack of knowledge about arthritis and hospital environment.
9. Worried about how she will care for her family.

Those statements spell out the exact nature of Mrs. Leigh's problems. Plans could now be made with and for Mrs. Leigh to alleviate them. Can you see the difference between these problems and the ones stated in the preceding list?

Note another approach to nursing care plans which seems generally to be ineffective. It amounts to stating the patient's need for some particular nursing task as the problem, e.g. needs to be fed. This may in truth be so but if that is placed on the problem side of the care plan, what is the nursing approach going to be?

Problem	*Approach*
patient to be fed	feed the patient

That indeed seems ridiculous to write down, and hence nurses say "nursing care plans are a waste of time." This approach fails to get at either the patient problem or the nursing problem. In addition it fosters task-centered nursing. It does not encourage the nursing team to thoroughly assess the patient's needs or to formulate nursing objectives. If, on the other hand, the nursing team asks "what is the patient's need disturbance or problem?" and, once having determined this, goes on to ask "what must we do to correct or prevent the disturbance?" then a meaningful plan is more likely to be developed.

Compare the following two patients:

(a) Mrs. Elvery, age 87, second hospital day. Diagnosis—anemia. Behavior: weak, tires easily, attention span very short, forgets where she is and who the nurses are. When her meals are brought to her she eats very little. Does not drink water or other fluids unless they are handed to her and she is given directions to drink. Talks to anyone who comes into her room. Sometimes her conversation is appropriate to the situation, sometimes it is not. Most of the time appears cheerful. Follows directions if they are given slowly and repeated often.

(b) Mr. Savoy, age 66, first hospital day. Diagnosis—anterior wall myocardial infarct. No chest pain since admission; no dyspnea; intelligent business man; alert and oriented; appears very concerned about his condition; appears well nourished; muscular body; no impairment in range of motion.

In both instances, the observed care plans stated under the heading "Problem" the statement—patient to be fed. In case (b) the patient's true problems are: decreased arterial blood supply to heart muscle and danger of cardiac rupture or failure. The nursing goal is: to decrease the work load of the heart (decrease the cardiac muscle's demands for oxygen) and to prevent further heart damage. The nursing plans for attaining these goals would most probably include feeding the patient as a means of minimizing activity, thereby providing rest for the heart.

In case (a) Mrs. Elvery's problems are: inability to maintain attention to eating her meals and inability to remember to take an adequate fluid intake. The nursing goals are: to assist the patient to maintain an adequate intake of food and fluids. The nursing plans for attaining these goals need not necessarily include the actual feeding of meals. Perhaps supervision at mealtimes would be sufficient and Mrs. Elvery could feed herself. Thereby the nursing team could also help Mrs. E. to maintain her sense of dignity and responsibility and also maintain activity. Perhaps a member of her family could be present at some mealtimes and could be alerted to realize her needs and thereby be better prepared to assist her when she is discharged. In this situation feeding the patient her meals would perhaps insure that she receives enough food and fluids. The other equally important goals would not be attained. It could happen that Mrs. E. would continue to be very inattentive while being fed. The nurse's aide might give up, not realizing the true problem and full range of desirable goals.

The nursing problem or goal cannot be formulated until the patient's problem is specifically identified. In a way, you might say that the patient's problem is where you are, the nursing goal is where you want to get to, the problem is how do you get from where you are to where you want to be.

Example:

Present situation: Mr. McGregor had had a myocardial infarct one week ago. He insists on doing everything for himself and has not been able to modify his activity pattern.

Desired goal: That Mr. McGregor accept his condition and modify his daily activities.

Nursing problem: How can we facilitate Mr. McGregor's acceptance of his condition and the changes it necessitates?

Example:

Present situation: Miss Le Leux's behavior expresses distrust of the nursing staff.

Desired goal: That Miss Le Leux learn that the nursing staff can be trusted.
Nursing problem: What experiences can we provide that will help Miss Le Leux to develop trust?
Example:
Present situation: Mr. Shoemaker has inadequate circulation to his right foot.
Desired goal: To increase circulation to the right foot.
Nursing problem: What measures can be employed to increase circulation to Mr. Shoemaker's right foot?

As with the patient's problem it is most important to state the nursing problem as specifically as possible.

SUMMARY

If assessment has been thorough and information validated, interpretation is not usually difficult. Failure to recognize the correct problem is usually due to inadequate assessment. In order to correctly interpret pertinent information, the nurse must have knowledge and be capable of utilizing that knowledge as well as the cognizance of relationships between facts. One method of problem identification is through the "recognition of a pattern." Simple problems are readily noted, whereas the more complex problems require more knowledge and facts for correct identification.

One may be misled into thinking that since the problem belongs to the patient, he should have the ability to correctly identify it. This is not always the case. He may only be aware of some part of the discomfort but the nurse needs to remember that the patient is the "key" person on the team denoting the problem.

All members of that team endeavor to do for the patient that which he cannot do for himself. Maintenance and promotion of as much independence as possible on the part of the patient are vital, as well as his understanding of his health problem and the means available to solve it.

A frequent source of difficulty for the team is differentiating between the patient's problem and the nursing problem. The nursing problem cannot be formulated *until* the patient's problem is identified. A rule of thumb to follow might be: how to get from where you are (patient's problem) to where you want to get (nursing problem).

Suggested Reading

Kozier, Barbara B. and DuGas, Beverly W., *Fundamentals of Patient Care*. Philadelphia: W. B. Saunders Co., 1967.

Orlando, Ida Jan, *The Dynamic Nurse-Patient Relationship*. New York: G. P. Putnam's Sons, 1961.

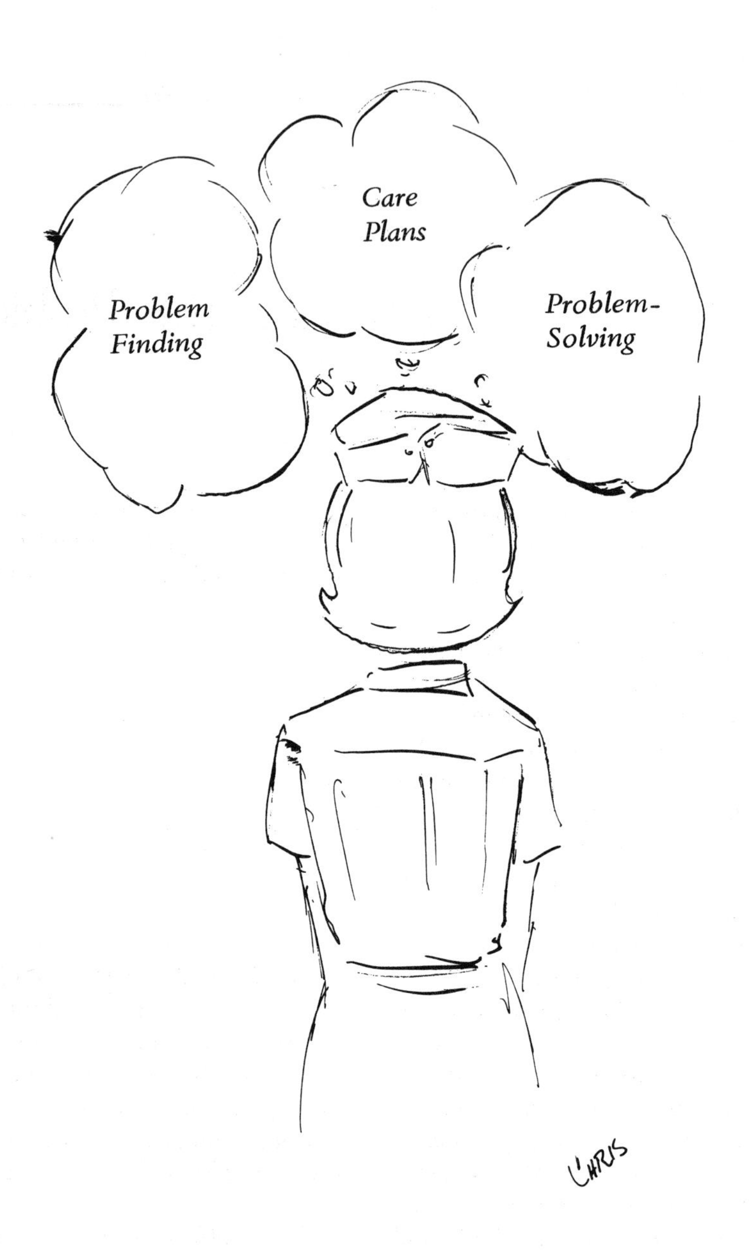
Care Plans
Problem Finding
Problem-Solving
CHRIS

Chapter 5

Solving the Problem

Although the entire process from assessment to evaluation is considered problem-solving, it is easy to see that the process divides quite naturally into two parts: The first part, problem-finding, which consists of:

1. Gathering information.
2. Examining the information.
3. Interpreting the information.
4. Identifying the problem(s).
5. Stating the problem(s).

The second part, problem-solving, consists of:

1. Developing alternatives.
2. Making a decision: choosing one of the possible methods.
3. Deciding on a plan of action.
4. Executing the plan.
5. Evaluating the results.

Essentially, problems are solved by reasoning, decision-making, and action. Repeating a statement from Chapter 1, it is man's ability for reflective thinking that enables him to solve difficult problems and thereby control his world. We know that animals solve problems and that a slight degree of reasoning may take place in the minds of some, but for most it is largely a matter of learned stimulus-response or random trial and error. Man sometimes solves problems this way but it is far from the most effective way.

Logical scientific methods must be used to effect solutions to problems and make wise decisions. Quite often it is impossible to be absolutely certain about the outcome of a particular action. Decisions should be based on the probabilities which you think the facts predict. For instance, you may test enough cases to predict that your premise is true 99% of the time or 80% of the time or 50% of the time. The degree of probability that you must have in order to act on a premise depends on the margin you have for error. If you are considering a new drug to be given to people you must have close to 100% probability that the drug is effective for what you say it is and that it is otherwise harmless. On the other hand, if you are predicting the effectiveness of a new deodorant you can be satisfied with, perhaps, 75% probability.

Actually what we really establish is a hypothesis. Hodnett says, "A hypothesis is an informed guess . . . that has some reasonable chance of being right. . . . When your hypothesis proves true enough of the time to convince you that it may be true all the time or with enough frequency to be of use, you indicate your increased certainty by calling it a theory. If it proves true invariably, you have discovered a law."[1] You can readily recognize how important it is for the nurse to develop correct thinking habits which lead to greater accuracy in decision-making. When she contracts with the public to give qualified nursing care in order to help solve their physical and mental health problems, she should be able to do so in an orderly manner. Health is too valuable, too precious. Decisions regarding its maintenance and restoration must be the product of a valid and accurate thought.

How the nurse goes about finding a solution is important. There are a number of ways which can be used to determine the method by which a solution can be achieved. These are the same methods you have used to solve your personal problems, and they shall be explored briefly and illustrated by their application to nursing situations. Notice the kinds of problems faced.

Krech and Crutchfield, in their book *Elements of Psychology*,[2] define two kinds of problems: "the quickly-solved problem" and "the difficult problem." Both kinds are encountered in nursing. In the first case, we see the problem and the solution almost simultaneously. Consider the following for an example:

Problem: How can we prevent Mrs. Rogers from falling out of bed while her eyes are covered following a cataract extraction? Solution: Put the bed rails up and arrange things where she can easily reach them.

In the case of the difficult problem the solution is not so easily perceived. The problem must be studied, looked at from various angles, and then solved through reasoning and/or experimentation. Consider this nursing problem: How can we facilitate Mrs. Jacob's adaptation to the limitations imposed by her cerebral vascular accident? The solu-

---

[1]Edward Hodnett, *The Art of Problem Solving* (New York: Harper & Row, Publishers, 1955).

[2]David Krech and Richard S. Crutchfield, *Elements of Psychology* (New York: Alfred A. Knopf, Inc., 1965), p. 359.

tion here is not so evident. This will require logical and creative thinking in addition to more knowledge.

Before moving on to discuss the methods which can be used to solve difficult problems, a few more words about the easy problem. There are, after all, many such problems in one's day-to-day experience in nursing.

In the early stages of a nursing career most problems seem difficult. However, through study, experience, and increased perception, many problems will be easily solved. You will find that if you continue to assess and identify the problem, particularly the most frequently met problems, solutions are readily found. A note of warning is necessary, however. Numerous successful solutions may possibly lead to a false sense of security for the advanced student or experienced nurse. Failure to follow conscientiously the steps outlined in previous chapters may have disastrous results. A too quick decision may lead to a habit of following the line of least resistance. Simply because you frequently meet with what appears to be the same type of problem does not necessarily mean the same solution will apply. No two problems however similar are exactly the same. Therefore, a solution too hastily or thoughtlessly chosen may bring about unfavorable results. The fact that no two problems are exactly alike is what makes problem-solving fascinating. Otherwise, much of nursing would result in routine boredom. Granted, there may be only a very limited number of possible solutions, carefully checking your choices should bring about desired results. Developing your ability to assess and identify a problem should increase your ability to select the best solution. Related to this is continued learning and experience, coupled with imagination and creativity. To add the last two ideas the nurse must be completely aware that she needs much knowledge and experience first.

Developing Alternatives

Up to this point the objectives of the process have been to determine the problem, define it, delimit it. Now you begin to plan your course of action. The first step is to consider your alternatives. *Mentally* you consider courses of action. By one course you may arrive at one solution, by another an entirely different one. It is necessary, therefore, to consider each possible action and possible solution or result. This may be accomplished by analogy, induction, deduction, reasoning, or use of a policy, rule, order, or procedure.

Analogy means to recognize similarities, correspondence, or parallelism. You see resemblance in one or more aspects about two things or two situations and reason that there are probably other similarities which are not as apparent. Therefore, you may hypothesize that what achieves success in one situation may also achieve success in a similar situation.

Consider the following situation: Mrs. Fujimoto had a hip pinning four days ago. She is a 72-year-old widow who had lived with her son and family for several years and been in good health. Her other married children live in the same community. She speaks English with difficulty. Her behavior indicates that she has retained many Japanese customs. Her progress since surgery has been satisfactory; however, she is not taking an adequate amount of food or fluids. All she will say is "I'm not hungry." The nursing problem is: "How can we get Mrs. Fujimoto to eat and drink sufficient amounts?"

The nurse recalls a similar situation a week ago. Mrs. Camponelli, a 76-year-old Italian woman, had also refused most of the food and fluids. She had had a small cerebral vascular accident (stroke), with only a slight weakness of the muscles on the left side of her body. She too spoke English with difficulty and retained many cultural mannerisms. The nurse had talked with her family about her likes and dislikes. She ate primarily Italian foods, highly seasoned. For beverages she liked wine and a special Italian blend of coffee. Between the dietitian and the family a diet was worked out. Sometimes the family brought in special meals that they had prepared. This, of course, meant that the family often spent the meal hour with their mother. Mrs. Camponelli began to eat an adequate diet.

These two situations parallel each other. Although there are a number of differences, there are also many similarities. It is reasonable to suppose that the two women may have similar reactions to hospital food and mealtime patterns. The nurse recognizes an analogy here. In addition, the nurse knows that eating habits are influenced by cultural background and family customs.

Induction is reasoning from the particular to the universal or that what is true of a sufficient number of instances or members of a class is true of all the instances or members. For example, if it is observed in a large number of cases that a drop of oil floats on water, we may reason that all drops of oil will float on water. It is through induction that the laws of the universe have been found. Edward Hodnett, in his very readable and interesting book, *The Art of Problem Solving,* says: "The aim of scientific induction is to arrive at general conclusions so invariably true that they may act as major premises for deductive inferences from there on."[3]

The validity of the induction demands that the instances observed be representative and that the studies be done under conditions which

[3]Hodnett, *op. cit.,* p. 135.

permit interpretation to be correct. In other words, we cannot say that dacron makes durable uniforms unless a sufficient number of uniforms have been made and worn. One or two uniforms could be the exception rather than the rule. In addition, these uniforms must all be subjected to the same kinds of wear and the observers must all follow the same rules for judgment.

Rarely, if ever, can complete testing be done. It would be impossible to test every drop of oil or every piece of dacron in existence. We must rely on a "sufficient" number. It is almost impossible to define this word. We can only explain it by saying that it is the number of instances which indicate a certain mathematical probability.

Deduction means that you reason from the universal to the particular or that what is true of all instances or members of a class is true of one instance or one member of that same class.

This is the type of reasoning which we use or attempt to use most of the time. Unfortunately we do not always make sure that the premise upon which we are acting is true. Many times we accept a generalization as always true. What is a generalization? It is an inference derived from observing a number of like situations and therefore thinking that the same inference applies to all situations.

There is a major premise, a minor premise, and a conclusion. The classic example is: A = C; B = C; A and B are equal.

For accuracy, the major premise must always be true. Here is a simple example of deductive reasoning: All persons in Mediville Hospital wearing an identification wristband are patients. Mr. Milburn, a person in Mediville Hospital, is wearing an identification wristband. Mr. Milburn is a patient. The statement beginning with "All persons" is called the major premise. It states a fact about a class of people. The same fact is true of Mr. Milburn. Therefore, you may conclude that Mr. Milburn is a member of the class described in the statement, i.e., he is a patient.

If the major or minor premise is not true, then the conclusions will not be true. This can be illustrated by the following: Pain is relieved by aspirin. Mr. Milburn has pain. Mr. Milburn's pain will be relieved by aspirin.

The major premise in this example is not always true. It is a generalization. Some kinds of pain for some people are relieved by aspirin, but not *all* types of *pain* for *all* people are relieved by aspirin.

A second hazard in the use of the deducting process is applying what *is* true of all members of a class to a member who *is not* of the class, as in the following example:

All alien persons disembarking from the Steamship must be interviewed by the Immigration Officer. Miss Rogers is disembarking from the Steamship. Miss Rogers must be interviewed by the Immigration Officer.

It turns out, however, that Miss Rogers is a citizen. It is true that all aliens must be examined, but Miss Rogers is not an alien.

Or consider this example:

In Valley Hospital, all children under 5 years of age must be in a crib. Three small children, Bobby, John, and Kevin, are admitted. They are all placed in cribs.

John is seven years old. He is small for his age. Here you have applied something which is true of all children under 5 to one who is over 5.

Another example of incorrect deduction is:

A person is at rest when he is in bed. Mrs. Golz is in bed. Therefore, Mrs. Golz is resting.

Studies now show that not all people rest while in bed. Some people rest more completely while sitting in a chair. Small children often wriggle around so in bed that they get less rest than if they were permitted to be out of bed playing at some simple game.

Induction and deduction are two methods of scientific reasoning. In the everyday course of events, however, we cannot have this degree of certainty and must rely on similar but less exact methods.

Reasoning from cause and effect or from effect to cause is an example of a less exact method and may also be used in combination with analogy. A hypothesis is then formulated. Since a hypothesis is a guess or supposition based on knowledge it has a reasonable chance of being correct. Since much of our knowledge is imperfect, our plan does not always work out as we expect. Nevertheless it may be the best that can be done at the time. Based on available information an informed guess is made. The plan is then tried and evaluated.

Continuing with our example, the nurse formulates the hypothesis that Mrs. Fujimoto will eat and drink if she has foods and fluids which she likes and if she has some of her family present at mealtimes. This is only a guess. There is no certainty that it will achieve the solution of the problem. It is, however, an *informed* guess and it has a reasonable chance of succeeding. On the other hand, Mrs. Fujimoto might tell the nurse why she is not eating. In this case, it is not necessary to draw an analogy. The nurse can reason from cause to effect. If food she does not like brings about the effect of not eating, then we can reason she will eat the food she likes. Note that in both situations the same course of action is selected. In one situation a course of action was selected by drawing an analogy to a similar situation. In the second, by reasoning from cause to effect.

When you reason from *cause* to *effect*, you are actually saying: "If I do . . . then . . . will happen." You postulate that a certain action (cause) will produce a certain effect. Surely you remember using this to solve some problems like "How can I get Mom to buy me a new dress for the dance?" or "How can I get Dad to let me use the car?" You figured that if you did the ironing or cleaned up your room all week or cut the lawn this would please your parents and they would react favorably to your request. You *caused* a certain effect.

Before relying on this method be sure that you establish that a relationship between the causative action and the expected effect does in fact exist. Also consider whether or not the effect you desire is the only one that could be produced by the action. The larger the number of possible effects that can be produced, the smaller the chances of producing the one effect you desire. Sometimes you may begin with the effects and try to deduce the cause. Once you have determined what is causing something you may be able to alter the cause and thereby change the effect (eliminating or alleviating the problem). This is one of the most commonly used methods in medicine and nursing. A nurse looks for clues (signs and symptoms) which tell her something about cause. A classic example is: redness, swelling, pain, and heat indicate an inflammatory process. Inflammation is known to be caused by injury (bacteriological, mechanical, chemical, or thermal). Suppose the doctor diagnoses the cause of the infection to be streptococcus. An antibiotic may be given which will cause the death of the organism and this will then be followed by other effects, e.g., wound healing.

One danger in reasoning from cause to effect is that of assuming that because one event follows another the first event caused the second. A patient receives a phone call. Five minutes after he hangs up he has an angina attack. One may then reason (incorrectly, perhaps) that the attack was caused by the nature of the phone conversation. Another example is that of the nurse who enters the pediatrics ward and finds two boys fighting. "Which one of you started this?" she inquires, assuming that one of the two boys started the fight, whereas in reality a third boy may have been the real instigator.

A common method of solving problems is the use of a *policy, rule, order, or procedure.* Webster defines a policy as "a definite course or method of action selected (by a government, group or individual) from among alternatives and in light of given conditions to guide and usually determine any future decisions."[4]

---

[4] Webster's Third International Dictionary, (Chicago: Encyclopaedia Britannica, Inc., 1966), p. 1954.

All health agencies have policies which guide nursing action. The nursing profession plays a large part in helping formulate these policies. The nurse must familiarize herself with the policies of the agency which employ her.

For many patient problems the physician writes a specific order for action. For many nursing actions procedures have been established to serve as a guide to performance.

It must be remembered that policies and procedures are intended to guide decision-making and action, not to make decisions. One must guard against inflexibility and the routine use of these without clearly understanding their meaning and purpose. Unfortunately, in some institutions, policies and routines which have lost their usefulness are still employed. These more often cause than solve problems.

Sometimes, even when you have used all these methods, the problem seems unsolvable. Then you must try to look at it from a different viewpoint. If you cannot fulfill all the requirements necessary to achieve your goal you may have to change or modify the goal, tackle a slightly different problem, or perhaps only one part of the total problem.

Hodnett offers three techniques for restructuring the problem:[5]

1. Change of point of view.
2. Permissible change of objective.
3. Rearrangement of the elements.

Suppose that your goal is to get Mr. Alenburg up in a chair three times a day. He is 82 years old, 6' 2" in height, and weighs 190 lbs. He has had a stroke and is totally paralyzed on the right side. Most of the time he is confused and resists attempts to move him. It takes three or four people to lift him, and no sooner is he up he calls to be put back in bed. The nursing staff is exasperated. But let's look at the problem in another way. Let's phrase the objective a little differently: to place Mr. Alenburg in an upright position and to change the pressure points on his back.

At mealtime Mr. Alenburg could be placed in a sitting position on the side of the bed with support. Since someone must assist him to eat, a nurse or aide would be at the bedside during this time. He eats slowly and the mealtime activity distracts him. In this way the objective can be achieved. Hodnett says, "The only problem you are likely to solve is the one you *think* you have to solve."[6] If you continue to see your problem as "How can we get Mr. Alenburg up into a chair?" you will work only on that problem. On the other hand, an answer may be found ". . . by altering the conditions of the problem in a permissable way."[7]

---

[5]Hodnett, *op cit.*, p. 86.
[6]*ibid.*, p. 103.
[7]*ibid.*, p. 105.

Deciding on a Plan of Action

Each step described thus far is essential to the formulation of your plan of care. Nevertheless, this is a step in and of itself. It requires time in seconds, minutes, or hours, depending on the number and kind of problems presented. It involves the following:

1. Examining the methods chosen.
2. Identifying the specific actions which must be taken.
3. Identifying the knowledge and skills necessary to carry out the action safely.
4. Deciding which team members are qualified to carry out the actions involved.
5. Estimating the time required to carry out the actions.
6. Estimating the factors which may facilitate or hinder the execution of the actions.
7. Identifying the modifications or adaptions which must be made for the individual patient.
8. Identifying the equipment which will be needed.
9. Determining how much time can be allotted for the care of this given patient (considering the time needed for the care of other patients under the care of this nurse or nursing team).
10. Determining which problems should receive priority.

All of the above must be considered regardless of whether the nurse is dealing with one simple problem for one patient or a number of complex problems for several patients. You learn to formulate nursing plans by working out simple problems under guidance. As you gain nursing knowledge and experience with nursing problems you will find that you can plan for more complex problems and a larger number of problems concurrently.

For the benefit of the beginning student try planning nursing care related to simple nursing problems in a simple nursing situation.

Nursing Situation: It is 8 a.m. You (the student) are assigned to care for two patients. You must complete your assignment, give a report to the Team Leader, and leave the unit at 11:00 a.m. to return to the college for classes. You cared for Mrs. Cosgrove yesterday and are aware of the information already compiled about these patients by the nursing team. You have been on the unit since 7:00 a.m. and have visited both patients and reviewed their charts and care plans.

Patient No. 1: Mrs. Cosgrove, age 43, is three days postabdominal hysterectomy. She has been taking a full liquid diet in adequate quantities. (Medical Plan permits diet as tolerated.) Demerol 50 mg. I.M. has been given q 6-8 hrs. during the last two days for typical incisional pain. She received her last dose at 2 a.m. and slept thereafter. Now she has moderate abdominal distention, abdomen is soft. She is experiencing intestinal cramps and is unable to expel flatus. The medical plans permit her to be up as much as she desires. Says she was up briefly 4 times yesteday. She walked about in her room and went to the bathroom (located in her room).

Patient No. 2: Mrs. Romano, age 68, is to go to surgery at 11:00 a.m. for a vaginal hysterectomy. She was admitted yesterday at 2:30 p.m. The evening and night teams compiled the following information: widow for 7 years, lives alone two houses away from her daughter, Gina, and family; has not been hospitalized since the birth of her last child thirty-five years ago; has 5 children living and well. Mrs. Romano went to her doctor one month ago for her yearly physical. The pelvic examination revealed a fibroid tumor. The medical examination revealed no other physical problem. The doctor advised surgery and she consented. A general inhalation anesthesia will be given.

The evening nurse recorded that she explained the preparation that will be carried out prior to surgery (evening enemas, the withholding of food and fluids after midnight, the skin preparations, the medications, etc.) and offered to answer any questions. Mrs. Romano has asked no questions and has made no comment about the surgery to the nurses or nurse aides although both spent time talking with her and provided opportunity for her to talk about these things if she had wished to do so. She appears calm. There are three religious pictures taped to her bed. She is frequently observed with her rosary in her hands and appears to be praying. The priest visited her at 7 a.m. and she received communion. She received nembutal 100 mg. at 12:00 a.m. and slept until 6:00 a.m. She is to receive Demerol 75 mg., Phenergan 25 mg., and Scopolamine 0.3 mg. at 10:00 a.m.

Imagine now that you or you and the team identify the nursing problems either mentally or in discussion. You have considered what methods are available to you for solution of the nursing problems and have selected the actions you will take. The following represents what might take place mentally:

Mrs. Cosgrove's Problems:

1. Decrease peristalsis (possibly due to surgery, anesthesia, diet and exercise restrictions) and inability to expel flatus.
2. Lack of comfort—intestinal and incisional pain.

Nursing Problems for Mrs. Cosgrove:	*Nursing Actions Selected*:
a. To promote peristalsis and expulsion of flatus, to decrease intestinal irritation.	Administer Harris Flush (for which there is a p.r.n. physician's orders).

Nursing Problems for Mrs. Cosgrove:	*Nursing Actions Selected*:
	Increase the amount of time she is up walking, increase number of activities she performs for herself.
	Restrict ice water and gas-forming liquids.
b. To maintain healthy skin and teeth and prevent body and mouth odors.	Assist Mrs. C. to wash skin with soap and water and brush teeth after meals.
c. To maintain fluid and caloric intake.	Provide fluids for Mrs. C. Explain the importance of fluids.
d. To meet patient's appetite and food desires.	Order a regular diet as soon as she begins to expel flatus.

Mrs. Romano's Problems:

1. None evident.

Nursing Problems for Mrs. Romano:	*Nursing Actions Selected*:
a. To prepare her respiratory tract and nervous system for anesthesia.	Administer pre-op medication at 10:00 a.m.
b. To prevent nausea and vomiting during and postanesthesia.	Withhold food and fluids.
c. To prevent injury during surgery.	Instruct patient to remove her dentures, hairpins, and religious medal at 9:45. Check that she does so.
d. To prevent injury to the bladder during surgery and prevent bladder distention following surgery.	Have patient void between 8-10 a.m.
e. To allow Mrs. R. to express her feelings about the surgery if she wishes to.	Permit Mrs. R. to talk; use reflective techniques of communication.
f. To assist Mrs. R. to learn how to do the post-op breathing exercises and cough.	Teach her how to do breathing exercises and coughing.

(You will note that even when there are no patient problems present or apparent there are still nursing problems. That is because nursing care is necessary to maintain health or prevent disturbances as well as to correct problems.)

Now you are ready to formulate a plan of care for each patient. But, you say, is that not the nursing plan which is outlined above? No, it is not. It is only part of the process. It represents assessment, problem--finding, the choosing of methods to solve the problems. What you are going to do now is make up a plan by which these chosen actions can be carried out in a manner and order which suits the individual needs and desires of both patients, but does not neglect the need or desires of either one. Review the facts listed for formulating your plan of care.

What are the specific actions which must be carried out:

1. Gathering of equipment to give Harris Flush.
2. Administration of Harris Flush.
3. Disposing of equipment.
4. Explanation of procedure to patient.
5. Instruction of Mrs. C. regarding activity.
6. Instruct Mrs. C. and other team members about the kinds of fluids to provide.
7. Observe Mrs. C.'s abdomen and/or question her about expelling flatus.
8. Prepare equipment and supplies for bathing and oral hygiene.
9. Wash legs, feet and back of Mrs. C.
10. Give Mrs. C. a back rub.
11. Gather clean linen and supplies.
12. Make bed.
13. Dispose of dirty linen and supplies.
14. Bring fluid nourishment to Mrs. C.
15. Call diet kitchen to order new diet.
16. Check diet list to be sure Mrs. R.'s diet is canceled.
17. Instruct Mrs. R. to void and remove dentures, etc.
18. Check that all the pre-op preparations are completed.
19. Visit Mrs. R., converse with her in a manner to facilitate expression of her feelings.
20. Demonstrate breathing exercises and how to cough.
21. Observe Mrs. R.'s deep breathing and coughing.
22. Explain reasons for breathing and coughing post-op.
23. Listen to Mrs. R.'s explanation.
24. Prepare the pre-op medication.
25. Give the medication.
26. Chart observations made and nursing care given for both patients.
27. Give an oral report to the aide and R.N. who will continue the patient's care after you leave.

What knowledge and skills are necessary to carry out these actions?

1. The size and temperature and contour of the rectum.
2. The position to place the patient in for a Harris Flush.
3. What a Harris Flush is and how to administer one.
4. What equipment is needed for a Harris Flush.
5. Where such equipment can be located.
6. What fluids produce gas in the intestines.
7. The general anatomy and psysiology of the skin and mouth.
8. What equipment is needed to bathe a patient and where it can be obtained in your situation.
9. How to order a new diet in your hospital.
10. The actions of Demerol, Phenergan and Scopolamine.

11. The safe range of dosage for each.
12. What the necessary preparations for surgery are in your particular situation.
13. Several techniques by which expression of feelings can be facilitated.
14. The reasons for breathing exercises and coughing after inhalation anesthesia.
15. One or two methods of teaching.
16. The correct way to breathe and cough after anesthesia and surgery.
17. The correct method of giving an intramuscular injection.

Would you need to be able to:

1. Give instructions.
2. Demonstrate an action.
3. Speak clearly.
4. Choose language which can be understood by the person to whom you are speaking.
5. Describe observation.
6. Write.
7. Hear.
8. Read.
9. Give an intramuscular injection.
10. Administer a Harris Flush.
11. Bathe another person.
12. Make a bed.
13. Measure liquid quantities.
14. Calculate dosage (add, subtract, multiply and divide, convert metric dose to apothecary and vice versa.

Do you or another member of the team have this knowledge and these skills? Which members have which knowledge and skills? To whom can you assign the various nursing actions chosen?

If you are assigned as a team leader you must evaluate your team members and make plans according to abilities of the team. There is no sense in making plans which none of the team is qualified to carry out.

What time will be required to carry out the actions you have chosen?

If you, the student, are going to carry out the plan you know you have three hours available. In this case there should be an adequate time if you organize well. Again, there is no sense to making a plan for which there is no time. If, for example, you plan to spend 45 minutes with Mrs. R. to permit her to talk with you, you will most likely run out of time and not complete your other plans.

What Equipment is Available or Obtainable

Plan within this framework. It would be fruitless to plan to instruct Mrs. R. by use of a film if no film is available or if the cost would be prohibitive.

In this way you can consider each factor on the list. Naturally this must be done mentally and rapidly. As your knowledge increases and you develop your powers of logical thinking you will find that this becomes almost second nature. One of the advantages of using this step-by-step process to find and solve problems is that you develop good habits in your thinking.

Once you have considered all the factors your plan might sound like this:

Mrs. Cosgrove:
1. Give Harris Flush immediately so that she can get some relief and perhaps be comfortable in time to take some breakfast.
2. Ask ward clerk to phone the kitchen and delay her breakfast till 9:00 a.m.
3. After Harris Flush instruct her to get up every 3-4 hours and walk around in the room and half way down the hall and back. Explain how activity promotes peristalsis. Instruct her to bathe the upper part of her body herself today and do other small personal activities.
4. Instruct her about not drinking ice water and gas-forming liquids. Explain which liquids are gas-forming.
5. Instruct her to inform you when she starts to expel gas and explain that you will then be able to increase her diet.
6. Assist her with her bath about 10:15-10:30 a.m. During this time reinforce instruction.

Mrs. Romano:
1. Between 9:00-10:00 a.m. spend time with Mrs. R. preparing her physically and emotionally for surgery. Do the demonstration of the breathing exercises and coughing at about 9:00 a.m. since this will focus on the surgery or perhaps encourage her to express her feelings.
2. Explain the reason for breathing exercises and coughing.
3. Use demonstration as teaching method. Have Mrs. R. return the demonstration.
4. After the demonstration have Mrs. R. state the reasons for the exercises in her own words.
5. Sit down with her while you talk to encourage discussion.
6. Check all the necessary pre-op preparations.
7. Give medication at 10:00 a.m.
8. Visit again at 10:30 a.m. to evaluate the effects of the medication.
9. Be with Mrs. R. when the orderly comes to transport her to surgery. Go to surgery with her if possible.

This appears very lengthy on paper but surely you can imagine how much more quickly it is done in reality.

Do you recognize the difference between choosing the methods for solving the nursing problems and actually formulating the plans? The first is more general, the latter is a specific adaptation of the methods to the individual and to your specific situation. The *plans* include the specific "hows" for the individual person.

This is the kind of planning that must go on minute to minute and hour to hour. Sometimes oral discussion with the team and verbal nursing orders are the most suitable, the most practical, and all that is necessary. The situation described above is such. There are other goals and problems which cannot be solved so quickly but which require the efforts of the nursing team on each shift. Then it is wise to have a written plan in order to insure consistency of approach and continuity of care.

SUMMARY

The first step in problem-solving is to determine what alternatives are available—then to make an hypothesis.

The alternatives or possible means of solution can be developed through the reasoning process known as induction and deduction.

Induction is reasoning from the particular to the universal; reasoning that what is true of a sufficient number of instances or members of a class is true of all the instances or members.

Deduction is reasoning from the universal to the particular or that what is true of all instances or members of a class is true of one instance or member of that same class.

An hypothesis may also be made by drawing an analogy, that is, to see resemblance in one or more aspects about two or more things or situations and reason that there are probably other similarities which are not as apparent.

The principle of cause and effect is also useful. If the cause can be established it may possibly be removed thereby eliminating the effect. On the other hand, observing the effects may enable you to determine the cause. Knowing the relationship between certain actions and the results is most useful in developing possible alternatives.

The next step is to make a decision. Choose the course of action which you believe will have the best chance for success. Knowledge and experience are the greatest assets.

The method you choose may be a direct action which can be immediately carried out. In some instances, however, the action chosen may be complex and it may be wise to formulate a plan by which to carry it out. Carefully analyze all the factors involved in the method of choice. Consider the kind and amount of equipment, time, and talent you have to work with.

The final step is evaluation.

Suggested Reading

Christman, Luther, "Assisting the Patient to Learn the 'Patient Role,'" *The Journal of Nursing Education,* January, 1967.

McDonald, Frederick J. and Harms, Mary T., "A Theoretical Model for an Experimental Curriculum," *Nursing Outlook,* Vol. 66, No. 8, 48-51.

McGregor, Frances C., "Uncooperative Patients: Some Cultural Interpretations," *American Journal of Nursing,* 67:88-91, 1967.

Paynick, Mary Louise, "Cultural Barriers to Nurse Communication," *American Journal of Nursing,* 64:87-90, February, 1964.

Reiter, Frances, "The Clinical Nursing Approach," *Nursing Forum,* Vol. V, No. 1, 1966, 41-42.

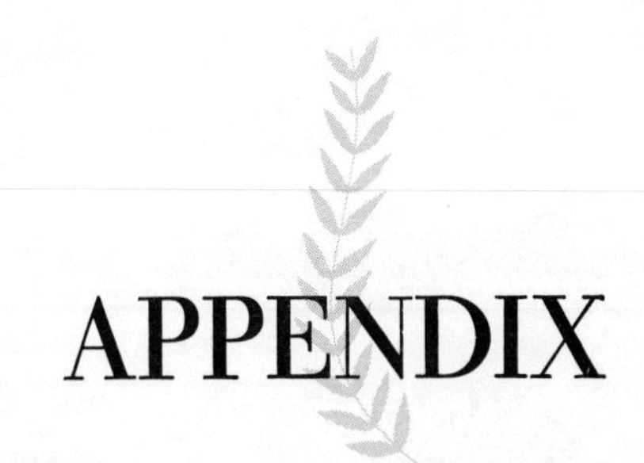

APPENDIX

Guide to Assessment of the Patient's Need for:
PHYSICAL COMFORT

To discover whether or not the patient has a problem or is in danger of developing a problem, seek answers to the following questions:

1. How old is the patient? How does this affect his skin and/or mouth condition?
2. What is the nature and extent of the patient's pathology? How does it affect his skin and/or mouth condition?
3. If surgery has been performed, what was the surgical procedure, where is the incision, how many days is it since surgery? What is extent of incision?
4. Does the skin appear clean?
5. Are there any special skin areas where accumulation of material is likely?
6. What does the patient consider comfortable?
7. What are the patient's usual hygiene habits?
8. When did the patient bathe last?
9. Is there a catheter in place?
10. Does the patient have bladder and bowel control?
11. Is there a dressing?
12. How many hours (out of 24) does the patient spend in bed?
13. What effect has the temperature and humidity on the patient?
14. Do his bed linens and clothes appear clean? Have an odor?
15. Do his teeth, tongue, and mouth appear clean?
16. Does he have dentures?
17. Is he taking fluids by mouth? Solid foods?
18. When did he brush his teeth last, or use a mouthwash?

The following are examples of problems you could discover by asking the above questions:

Discomfort.
Lack of personal cleanliness.
Lack of clean, comfortable environment.
Lack of clean clothes.
Accumulation of oils, sweat, dirt, bacteria, blood, drainage, etc., on skin.
Accumulation of food, bacteria, etc., in the mouth.

Guide to Assessment of the Patient's Need for:
SAFETY

To discover whether or not the patient has a problem or is in danger of developing a problem, seek answers to the following questions:

1. Is he rational? Is he oriented? Is he fully conscious?
2. Is he weak?
3. Is he emotionally upset? Might this interfere with his judgment?
4. Is he receiving any medication that might interfere with his consciousness, orientation, or judgment?
5. Are there factors in the environment which increase hazards: e.g., oxygen, room crowded with equipment, steam inhalators.
6. Does he have any motor impairment?
7. Does he have any sensory impairment? (particularly visual)
8. How old is he?
9. What is the number and virulence of the organisms in the environment?
10. Are there patients on the unit with known communicable organisms?
11. How great is the resistance of (or how susceptible is) the patient to infection? Are any of his lines of defense broken? Is his nutritional state satisfactory? Has he been ill for a long time?
12. Are there many vehicles available to transfer organisms from one person to another?
13. Does the patient have a retention catheter?
14. Has he had inhalation anesthesia?
15. Is he confined to bed for long periods of time?
16. Is he able to move about and turn in bed?

The following are examples of problems you could discover by asking the above questions:

Danger of injury.

1. Mechanical.
   e.g. Danger of falling out of bed.
2. Chemical.
   e.g. Danger of an acid burn; danger of incorrect drug dosage.
3. Thermal.
   e.g. Danger of burning self with cigarette.
4. Bacteriological.
   e.g. Danger of wound infection; danger of urinary tract infection.

Guide to Assessment of the Patient's Need for:

CORRECT BODY ALIGNMENT
SATISFACTORY BODY MECHANICS

To discover whether or not the patient has a problem or is in danger of developing a problem, seek answers to the following questions:

1. How old is the patient? How does this affect his skeletal-muscular system?
2. What is his pathology? Does it have a specific or even general effect on his muscular-skeletal system?
3. How does his emotional mood, his attitude, affect his posture?
4. Are there any environmental factors such as position of bed pillows, lighting, furniture, and space that affect his posture?
5. In what stage of his illness is he? Does this affect his posture or body mechanics?
6. Is he receiving any medication which affects his skeletal-muscular system?
7. Are there any other therapeutic measures which might affect his posture or body mechanics such as cobalt therapy, surgery, casts, traction?
8. What is his nutritional state? Does this have an effect?

The following are examples of problems you could discover by asking the above questions:

Incorrect posture (generally).
Internal and external rotation) of arm or leg.
Adduction or abduction) of arm or leg.
Plantar or dorsal flexion of a foot or hand.
Contracture (of any muscle or group of muscles).
Atrophy (of any muscle).
Loss of muscle tone.
Loss of impaired range of motion (of any joint).
A danger of—any of the above.

Guide to Assessment of the Patient's Need for:

A NUTRIENT SUPPLY FOR ALL BODY CELLS
A BALANCE OF FLUID INTAKE AND OUTPUT
A BALANCE OF ELECTROLYTES

To discover whether or not the patient has a problem or is in danger of developing a problem, seek answers to the following questions:

1. What kind and amount of food is the person *permitted* to eat (according to medical therapy)?
2. What kind and amount of food is the person *able to eat* (according to anatomy, physiology, pathology)?
3. What kind and amount of food *does* the patient eat?
4. What color are the nails, mucous membrane of mouth, conjunctiva?
5. Is the person underweight or overweight for height and age?
6. What is the patient's hemoglobin?
7. Are there factors which necessitate additional specific nutrients (wound healing, fractured bones, increased activity, increased metabolism)?
8. Are there factors which necessitate a decrease in amount of food (need for rest, decreased activity or metabolism)?
9. What are the patient's dietary habits?
10. What kinds of foods does he *like* or *dislike*?
11. What is his attitude toward food?
12. Are there factors interfering with appetite, eating, or digestion?
13. Is the person on solid foods in addition to liquids or is he on a liquid diet only?
14. Approximately how much fluid does the person take in a 24 hr. day?
15. By which route is the patient obtaining most of his fluid intake—oral, I.V., or gastrostomy?
16. What kinds of fluids does he like or dislike?
17. What kinds of fluids is he permitted by medical order?
18. Approximately what is the patient's 24 hr. output?
19. What are the results of blood chemistry studies (Na, K, Cl, B.U.N., etc.)?
20. Does he have any fluid restrictions?
21. Does he have adequate circulation to all body parts?

The following are examples of problems you could discover by asking the above questions:

Malnutrition (general)—Hunger.
Inadequate intake of specific nutrient (carbohydrates, protein, fats, vitamins).
Inadequate fluid intake—Dipphagia—Anorexia.

Guide to Assessment of the Patient's Need for: OXYGEN TO ALL BODY CELLS

To discover whether or not the patient has a problem or is in danger of developing a problem, seek answers to the following questions:

1. Is the respiratory rate within normal limits?
2. Are there factors present which could cause an increase or decrease in respiratory rate?
3. What is the temperature?
4. What is the pulse rate?
5. Is the rhythm normal? If not, what kind of irregularity is present?
6. What is the pathological process? Where is it?
7. What is the character of the respirations (breath sounds)? (deep/shallow, quiet/noisy)
8. Is the respiration affected by posture, by activity? To what degree?
9. Is the problem local or systemic?
10. Is there cyanosis? If so, where and to what degree?
11. Is there a change in skin temperature?
12. Is there pain? Where?
13. If O_2 is being administered, has it relieved the symptoms?
14. Is there an accumulation of respiratory secretions or danger of such?
15. Are there factors predisposing to accumulation of secretions? (posture, tracheotomy, anesthesia)
16. Is there danger of obstruction, or aspiration?
17. Is the patient coughing? Productive type, color, amount, viscosity?

The following are examples of problems you could discover by asking the above questions:

Dyspnea.
Hyperpnea.
Orthopnea.
Hypoxia (systemic).
Hypoxia (local-necrosis, ulceration).
Anoxia (local).
Accumulation of secretions in: nose.
pharynx.
trachea.
bronchioles.
lungs.
Obstruction of airway.

Guide to Assessment of the Patient's Need for:
ELIMINATION OF WASTE PRODUCTS AND FLUID

To discover whether or not the patient has a problem or is in danger of developing a problem, seek answers to the following questions:

1. Is the patient having regular bowel movements? If not, what factors are influencing regularity?
2. Is the patient able to expel flatus? If not, why?
3. Is the amount of defecation proportionate to patient's age?
4. What is the consistency of the stool (hard, dry, formed, loose, semi-loose, semi-liquid)?
5. What is the color of the stool (brown, tarry, bright red, clay colored)?
6. What factors are present which might be causing a deviation from normal color and consistency (medications, foods, pathology)?
7. Is the patient's abdomen distended? If so, to what degree?
8. If the stools are loose or liquid—how much, how often?
9. Is he able to voluntarily control defecation?
10. Is urinary output proportionate to intake?
11. What is the urine color, specific gravity?
12. Is the patient losing fluids by routes other than urinary tract (skin drainage)?
13. Is he able to exert voluntary control over urination?
14. What and where is the pathology? How does it affect elimination?
15. How old is the patient?
16. Did the patient have therapy which could affect elimination?
17. Did the patient have a general anesthetic?
18. How many hours or days postoperative?
19. Is defecation by other than normal route?

The following are examples of problems you could discover by asking the above questions:

Constipation
Diarrhea.
Abdominal distention.
Flatulence.
Retention of urine.
Suppression of urine (anuria).
Polyuria.
Oliguria.
Frequency.
Urgency.
Inability to control bowels or bladder.

Guide to Assessment of the Patient's Need for:

OPTIMAL ACTIVITY

(the best or most favorable degree of rest and exercise for the individual in his situation)

To discover whether or not the patient has a problem or is in danger of developing a problem, seek answers to the following questions:

1. What and where is the pathology?
2. How does the pathology affect the need for rest; for exercise?
3. How old is the patient?
4. How does age affect needs for rest and exercise?
5. How does the medical therapeutic plan affect the ability to rest or exercise?
6. Is the patient able to turn himself in bed?
7. Is he permitted to be out of bed?
8. Is he able to get out of bed without assistance? If so, how often does he get up? How long does he stay up?
9. When out of bed does he ambulate in room; beyond room?
10. Does he do most of his activities of daily living for himself?
11. If he is an "in-bed" patient, what activities is he able to do; what activities does he do? What activities should he be doing that he is not doing?
12. Is he receiving physical therapy? What kind? How often?
13. How many hours (in 24) does he sleep?
14. Does he require tranquilizers or sedatives?
15. What are his usual habits of rest and exercise?

The following are examples of problems you could discover by asking the above questions:

Inadequate rest or sleep.
Inadequate exercise—generally, or of a specific body part.

Guide to Assessment of the Patient's Need for:

RECOGNITION AND ESTEEM

To discover whether or not the patient has a problem or is in danger of developing a problem, seek answers to the following questions:

1. To what degree is his self-image threatened by his illness or hospitalization?
2. To what degree is his physical appearance altered by the pathology, surgery, or other therapy?
3. Does he talk about the affected body part or carefully avoid the subject?
4. Is he able to acknowledge the loss?
5. Does he take an interest in his appearance—clothes, make-up, hair? Or does he ignore these whereas prior to illness he had been concerned about appearance?
6. If a loss of body image has been sustained, are the patient's reactions following the normal pattern of grief?
7. Does any one stage in the grief process seem to be excessively prolonged?
8. Does the patient seem to be reacting to the real (objective) loss or to some special meaning the loss has for him?
9. How does the patient express his feeling about the events that are occurring during his illness?
10. Does he behave in an angry manner toward others and/or himself?
11. How does the patient express how he thinks others will feel about him?
12. Is he reacting to how he thinks others feel about him or to how they really feel?
13. How does he identify himself? (As Bob Jones, an engineer, just another patient, or nobody)?
14. What is his occupation? Education? Intelligence?
15. Does he assume the responsibility for which he has the intellectual potential?
16. Is he at home or in a hospital?
17. If he is in the hospital, is it for a long-term or short-term stay? What kind of a hospital is it—city, county, veterans, state, private?
18. Does the hospital permit him to wear his own clothes? Is he permitted to wear clothes other than pajamas and bathrobe?
19. Is he permitted to have personal belongings and display them in his unit? If so permitted, *does* he do this?
20. What is the family constellation? What is the patient's place and role in it?
21. In what way does his illness, hospitalization, or surgery influence his place and role in the family?
22. Does the patient's illness, hospitalization, or surgery affect the masculine or feminine image?

23. Do the physical limitations imposed by the illness or surgery prevent him from carrying out the usual activities of daily living?
24. If he must have help with bathing, dressing, elimination, ambulatory, eating, what is his reaction?
25. Has he had an opportunity to talk about his reactions to and feelings about these activities?

The following are examples of problems you could discover by asking the above questions:

Total or partial loss of self-esteem (self-worth, self-image, self-concept.

Loss of feeling of individuality.

Loss of individual identity.

Guide to Assessment of the Patient's Need for:

PSYCHOLOGICAL COMFORT
(Security, Freedom from Threat)

To discover whether or not the patient has a problem or is in danger of developing a problem, seek answers to the following questions:

1. Is his pulse and respiratory rate increased?
2. Is he perspiring (without any objective cause)?
3. Does he complain of frequent thirst?
4. Has he developed diarrhea and/or frequency (without pathologic cause)?
5. Has he lost his appetite or is he extremely hungry?
6. Does he have difficulty concentrating on events, conversation, or tasks at hand?
7. Is his behavior pattern disorganized?
8. Is he restless? Is he unable to sleep?
9. Does he frequently pace about the room or corridors?
10. Are his hand movements "nervous"? Is he constantly rearranging small objects about him, biting his nails, fussing with hair or clothes?
11. Has he just been admitted? Has he ever been hospitalized before? Has he ever been in this hospital before?
12. Does he know his diagnosis? Or is he awaiting the outcome of diagnostic studies?
13. Is his prognosis favorable or unfavorable? Does he know?
14. Is he to have surgery (in the O.R.) or any surgical procedures (in his room)? If so, what kind?
15. Has he had an opportunity to discuss his feeling with anyone?
16. Has anyone answered his questions regarding his illness, hospitalization, or surgery?
17. What is his age? How does this influence his reaction to illness and/or hospitalization?
18. Is his hospitalization sudden or was it planned? Was there opportunity to make arrangements for family and job?
19. Is he hospitalized near his home?
20. What is the family constellation? What is the patient's place and role in it?
21. Do family and friends visit regularly? Do they seem able to communicate adequately with one another? Do they seem mutually concerned?
22. Does the family understand what is happening? Have they had an opportunity to discuss their feelings?
23. Is he about to be discharged? Has he had an opportunity to discuss his reactions?
24. Has anyone discussed his care at home with the family?
25. Does he have insurance to cover his illness or other financial resources?

26. Is his job endangered?
27. Does he seem compatible with his roommate?
28. Is the roommate's behavior disturbing in any way?

The following are examples of problems you could discover by asking the above questions:

Anxiety.
Fear.

Guide to Assessment of the Patient's Need for:

MOTOR AND SENSORY FUNCTION

To discover whether or not the patient has a problem or is in danger of developing a problem, seek answers to the following questions:

Motor Function:

1. How old is the patient? Does his age affect his neurological and muscular development?
2. What is the nature and extent of the pathology? How does the pathology affect motor function?
3. Can the patient voluntarily contract all skeletal muscles? (e.g., can he flex the leg, extend the arm, grasp with his hand, smile, frown, extend tongue, etc.?)
4. If there is loss of voluntary control, is it a partial or total loss? If partial, attempt to determine degree of loss.
5. Does he have bladder and bowel control?
6. Is there loss of involuntary (reflex) movement?
7. Are the muscles of the affected part limp or more tense than normal?
8. Is there atrophy of the involved muscles?
9. Is there any loss of ability to speak or write? Is speech slow, monotonous, or slurred?
10. Are pupils round, equal? Do they react to light? Can eye movements be controlled and coordinated?
11. Are there convulsive movements of the whole body or a part of the body?
12. If there are convulsive movements, what type are they? How do they begin? Where do they begin?
13. Are there any disturbances in manner of walking (atapic gait, scissor gait, spastic gait, shuffling gait)?
14. Are there involuntary movements? What kind (fine, coarse, slow, rapid, intentional)?
15. Does the therapy in any way affect his motor abilities (e.g., surgery, drugs, application of casts)?
16. Is his skeletal system intact?

Sensory Function:

1. How does the pathology or injury affect his sense organs (eyes, ears, skin, nose, tongue)?
2. Does the therapy in any way impair his sensory function (e.g., brain surgery, eye surgery, dark glasses, drugs which dilate the eyes)?
3. Is the loss of sight, hearing, smell and taste total or partial? If partial, attempt to determine degree of loss.
4. Is there a loss of touch perception? To what degree? To any special kind of stimuli–sharp, dull?
5. Is there a loss of temperature perception?

6. Is there a loss of the ability to perceive extent or direction, or weight of movement, position in space?
7. Is there any unusual sensibility to sensory stimuli?

The following are examples of problems you could discover by asking the above questions:

Motor Problems:

Inability to move (the whole body or any part of it).
Impairment (or partial loss) of ability to move body or body part.
Inability to speak, i.e., to verbalize words (emissive aphasia).
Inability to write (agraphia).
Defects or distortions in voluntary movement (dyskinesia), tremors, convulsions, disturbances in gait, mystagnus.

Sensory Problems:

Loss or impairment of sight, hearing, smell, taste.
Insensibility to sensory stimuli.
Hypersensitivity to sensory stimuli.
Distortions of sensitivity (crawling sensations on skin, tingling, painfulness of sensation which is not normally painful).
Auditory aphasia—inability to understand and repeat words.

Sensory–Motor Problems:

Kinetosis—motor sickness.
Dyskinesthesia—inability or disturbance in ability to position and direction of body and body parts.
Vertigo.

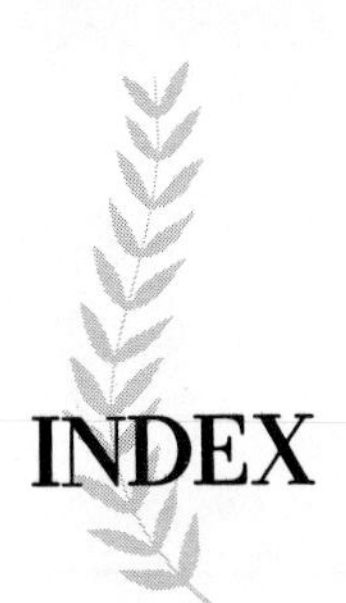

INDEX